1   Introduction

Our soul and spirit combine in our physical bodies to make us who we are. This is a book about living but when we talk about the soul and our spirit, there also needs to be a conversation around what they mean at the time of our death. Some of this book refers to an ancient Tibetan book written in the eighth century, The Tibetan Book of the Dead. Before the eighth century information in, it was an oral tradition passed down by shamans and from which its heritage stems. But its tradition and information go much further back and are based on prehistoric shamanic intelligence. Ancient knowledge became part of the Bon religion, which is still practised today. When Buddhism entered Tibet, Bon, and the Tibetan Book of the Dead became part of Buddhist discipline, helping to make Tibetan Buddhism unique.

In the Tibetan worldview, there is no destructive death at the end of life as it is in the west. Instead, there is reincarnation, rebirth, and a transition into a new life. What we do in this life, the good and bad deeds, or Karma influence the rebirth of our soul and how it will continue to seek enlightenment.

ccording to Tibetan tradition, after death and before one's next birth, when one's consciousness or soul is not connected to a physical body, it passes through several states. Some are like those reported by people who have had a Near-Death Experience. Soon after the Buddha's passing, it was recognized that we experience different states of existence each day of our lives and after we die. These intermediate, or liminal, states are called Bardos. Our waking life is a Bardo state; our dreaming at night is a Bardo state, if or when we meditate, that is another Bardo state.

This book is part of the Shaman series, which includes broad introductions to shamans and shamanism and concentrates on the Soul and the Spirit, together with the beliefs and rituals that surround both and why they differ.

Reiki, Shamanism, and essential loving mysticism are complementary to our:

- YouTube video series, "Reiki and Shamanism,"

- "The Shaman Podcast" on iTunes, Spotify, Google Podcasts, iHeart Radio, Stitcher, Tunine, Deezer and more.

Connect with our Private Facebook group to learn more about Reiki. Click here.

Subscribe to our newsletter to learn more about Reiki and Shamanism. Click here

Enjoy.
Mark Ashford, MSc,
Usui Tibetan Reiki Master and Teacher
https://www.markaashford.com

information@markaashford.com

Soul and Spirit

2 Table of contents

3   Table of figures

4   The Body, Soul, and Spirit

The physical structure and material substance of an animal or plant, living or dead[1]

4.1   Human Body

The human body is the material and physical structure of a human being. It is composed of many cells that together create tissues and organ systems. They ensure homeostasis and the viability of the human body. [2]

It comprises a head, neck, trunk (which includes the thorax and abdomen), arms and hands, legs and feet. [3]

The study of the human body involves anatomy, physiology, histology, and embryology. The body varies anatomically in known ways. Physiology focuses on the systems and organs of the human body and their functions. Many systems and mechanisms interact in order to maintain homeostasis, with safe levels of substances such as sugar and oxygen in the blood. [4]

The body is studied by health professionals, physiologists, anatomists, and by artists to assist them in their work.[5]

It is the physical entity we interact with, on the subway, in the grocery store, at work, in love, or when we are in conflict.

The physical body is what we find attractive in a man or woman until we know the person better. It is the physical body that creates limitations, such being confined to a wheelchair, and it grants gifts, such as being artistic or proficient and admired in sports. These gifts and limitations are part of the boundary to the learning experience of the soul and in which the spirit must work.

4.2   Other Bodies

Human beings are not the only physical beings that have a body; animals, plants, and cells also have bodies.

Animals are multicellular eukaryotic organisms that form the biological kingdom Animalia. With few exceptions, animals consume organic material, breathe oxygen, can move, can reproduce sexually, and grow from a hollow sphere of cells, the blastula, during embryonic development. Over 1.5 million living animal species have been described—of which around 1 million are insects—but it has been estimated there are over 7 million animal species in total. Animals range from 8.5 millionths of a meter to 33.6 metres (110 ft). They have complex interactions with each other and their environments, forming intricate food webs. The kingdom Animalia includes humans, but in

---

[1]

[2] Wikipedia, HumanBody.
[3] Ibid.
[4] Ibid.
[5] Ibid.

colloquial use the term animal often refers only to non-human animals. The scientific study of animals is known as zoology.[6]

When we consider the cellular world, cellular respiration[7] is a guide as to the activity in the cell and the world within and without the cell and the life process taking place in it, which is a mirror of what is taking place in human and animal bodies.

The body is a complex organization of cells, bones, and connective tissues which take together inhabited physical space, whether alive or dead, even when cremated. The body's ashes take up space. If you reach out with your index finger, you can touch your body and that of other human beings and animals and you can use tools such as microscopes to study other life forms.

4.3   The Soul

The soul[8] in many religious, philosophical, and mythological traditions is the incorporeal[9] essence, the nonmaterial form of a living being. Soul or psyche comprises the mental abilities of a living being: reason, character, feeling, consciousness, memory, perception, thinking, etc. Depending on the philosophical system, a soul may be mortal or immortal.

The soul includes other forms of incorporeal essence. It includes our emotions, our will to do something, or not. Our thoughts and our feelings. It is through our soul that we sense hurt and suffering and pleasure and enjoyment. Our soul experiences the energy and drive, or discouragement of external stimuli and how we respond to it.

When we collect all these incorporeal reactions to stimulus, we come to life and others around us, human or animal, react to us. Some people have good relations with other humans and animals; some do not. This outward expression of the soul becomes what we and others describe as our personality.
To a great extent, the expression of our personality is reinforced by repeated, similar reactions from those around us. External shocks and changes can change our personality. The sudden loss of a loved one, human or animal, can be so fundamental that other aspects of our soul come to the surface that had previously not had expression.

Reincarnation[10] is the philosophical or religious concept that the non-physical essence of a living being, the soul, starts a new life in a different physical form or body after biological death. It is also called rebirth or transmigration.[11] Through different lifetimes, the soul gathers unique experiences and it expresses Karma, which it carries from one to another, over and over an effort to seek enlightenment and ascendance.

4.4   Spirit

---

[6] Wikipedia, Animal.
[7] CellularRespiration.
[8] Soul.
[9] Dictionary.com, Incorporeal.
[10] http://healerofheartsandminds.com, Reincarnation,PastLives,SufferingandtheBible,aShaman'sViews.
[11] Wikipedia, Reincarnation.

What we call a Spirit[12] [13] [14] is also incorporeal. If the soul exists within us and gathers experience through lifetime after lifetime, then in each life, it is the spirit that gives expression to the soul's gained knowledge and our thoughts and mental capabilities. It expresses personality, knowledge, and wisdom. It is what moves our body.

Because a person's soul is a combination of all that it has experienced before in previous lives, plus our logic, thoughts, emotions and experiences in this life, which are driven by the spirit, that spirt cannot continue after the body's physical death. Its role was to help the soul experience a lifetime of physical existence. At the moment of death, when the soul leaves the corporeal body to be reincarnated, the spirit's work is complete, and it does not continue.

---

[12] Spirit.
[13] Dictionary.com, SpiritDefinitionofSpirit.
[14] Longman Dictionary of Contemporary English, SpiritMeaningofSpirit.

5 Difference Between Spirit and Soul

The soul and the spirit are energy beings connected to the physical body during its lifetime. Collectively, they are the "people" we experience at work, on the train, and as a driver of the cab, we are travelling in.

As energy beings, connected to a physical body, we must see all three as part of nature and susceptible to the actions of spirits in nature that can directly affect the life energy of an individual, including their immune system, thoughts, and private energy field. When there is an imbalance, either within the person or the person and their natural surroundings, it is necessary to engage an expert healer, a shaman, to re-establish the primordial harmony existing between the person and nature. Rebalancing the harmony of an individual's soul and spirt affects a cure and a healing.

Death brings the soul to the six Bardo states, and the process of rebirth. The spirit is not immortal, unlike the soul. When the soul reincarnates into a new life, it encounters a new spirt that will grow from birth through to adulthood with the physical body. At death, the spirit ceases to exist along with the physical body it has used to help the soul gather experiences.

It is important to remember that when the soul, consciousness, leaves the physical body, it may remain for a while around the body, in a favourite room, or around a favourite person without connecting to the dead body. When the soul leaves its body, it will see it and not connect with the meaning of it. This sets it apart from the Out of Body Experiences, where there is a necessary connection to what is still a physically living body. The connection of soul, spirit, and body disappears in the dissolution stage of dying.

Death is usually a very emotional environment.

People are crying, expressing themselves emotionally, naming the body, recalling his life and his qualities, his virtues, etc. Maybe competitors or people who did not like him are criticizing, complaining, and glad that he is no longer physically around. But all of this, the good and the bad, are gone. Dissolution has reset the counter to the memories and experiences of consciousness.

A Shaman will be called if the emotions of those who knew the soul in physical form are so strong, they are holding the soul to the physical realm, causing it to reconnect with them. Later, if the soul disconnects but does not complete the process of rebirth, it may wander the physical realm, connecting to people with which it has no purpose, but may sometimes cause injury to those living souls and consciousness.

A soul in the Bardo may encounter difficulties with reincarnation, or the karma of the soul may be such that the soul resists reincarnation because of the prospect of suffering it perceives to be waiting for it in a new life. The family of the deceased may engage a shaman to assist a soul in the Bardo with its reincarnation if they are aware of the soul's difficulties, or some other circumstance, such as a death by accident, or suicide causes a soul to remain on the physical plane. No family member desires the intervention of departing a soul or it reappearing in their lives.

A soul that remains in the Bardo and tries and influences a new soul not to reincarnate or to accept a bad reincarnation is known as spirits, and may be a "friendly spirit," or a "malevolent or dark spirit."

Because these souls have not reborn, and are interacting with different souls in the process of their reincarnation or through their actions trying to return to the physical realm they are referred to as "spirits" rather than souls, and often perceived or believed to be dark spirits and take on the role of demons and evil deities.

Other spirits, those of enlightened beings, Buddhas, prophets, or spirits of souls with good karma, may purposefully not reincarnate to help other souls and provide information and protection to the shaman, as the latter connects with the upper, lower, and intermediate [physical] worlds on behalf of humans, who cannot do this.

To the shaman, his/her universe includes an upper, middle and lower realm where spirits exist, along with the spirits of ancestors who must be understood and persuaded to help a soul in its current physical incarnation. In these realms, Shaman encounter demons, and dark spirits when they journey into them and into the Bardo to assist souls with their rebirth or to retrieve a soul when it has been lost or part of it has been stolen, and to promote healing for a client. The shaman's protective helping spirits are those souls that have chosen not to be reborn but to be helping and supportive spirits.

How and why a soul did not cross over and has been in this state for many hundreds of years comes down to the Karma of the soul when it entered the intermediate state between life and rebirth.

6   Reincarnation

6.1   Etymology

Bardo—Tibetan—Bar does thos grol translates as: [15]

1. Bardo "intermediate state," "transitional state," "in between states," "liminal state," which is synonymous with the Sanskrit antarabhāva. Valdez: "Used loosely, the term 'Bardo' refers to the state of existence intermediate between two lives on earth." Valdez: "[The] concept arose soon after the Buddha's passing, with several earlier Buddhist groups accepting the existence of such an intermediate state, while other schools rejected it."

2. Thos grol: "liberation," which is synonymous with the Sanskrit word bodhi, "awakening," "understanding," "enlightenment," and synonymous with the term nirvana, "blowing out," "extinction," "the extinction of illusion."

3. In Tibetan Buddhism, Bardo is the central theme of the Bardo Thodol literally Liberation Through Hearing During the Intermediate State, the Tibetan Book of the Dead

6.2   Origins.

In Tibetan tradition, the Bardo Thodol, Liberation Through Hearing During the Intermediate State — The Tibetan Book of the Dead was composed in the 8th century by Padmasambhava, written by his primary student, Yeshe Tsogyal, buried in the Gampo hills in central Tibet and subsequently discovered by a Tibetan terton, Karma Lingpa, in the 14th century.[16]

In some schools of Buddhism, Bardo, antarabhava, or chuu is an intermediate or liminal state between death and rebirth—reincarnation. Reincarnation into another life, as a different being, is the philosophical or religious concept that the non-physical essence of a living being starts a new life in a different physical form or body after biological death. It is also called rebirth or transmigration.[17]

Bardo or Bardo Thodol is a concept which arose soon after the Buddha's passing, with several earlier Buddhist groups accepting the existence of such an intermediate state, while other schools rejected it.
In Tibetan Buddhism, Bardo is the central theme of the Bardo Thodol[18]; literally Liberation Through Hearing During the Intermediate State, in the west, Bardo Thodol is known as the Tibetan Book of the Dead.[19] The Tibetan Book of the Dead is a Lamest book of counsel, probably influenced by Bon shamanism. The Tibetan text should guide one through the experiences consciousness has after death, in the Bardo, the interval between death and the next rebirth. The text also includes chapters on the signs of death and rituals to undertake when death is closing in or has taken place.

---

[15] Wikipedia, BardoThodol.
[16] http://donlehmanjr.com/, TheTibetanBookoftheDead.Pdf.
[17] https://en.wikipedia.org/wiki/The_City_of_God, TheCityofGod.
[18] Britannica, BardoThöDolTibetanBuddhistText.
[19] Wikipedia, Bardo.

One common error with the Tibetan Book of the dead is that it is not whispered into the dying person's ear! In Tibetan Buddhist practice, the Tibetan Book of the Dead is used during life by those who want to learn to visualize what will come after death.

After physical death, it is the tribal shaman, a psychopomp or soul-guide who accompanies the soul of the dead person on their hard path during the forty-nine days of the intermediate state between death and rebirth.[20]

According to Tibetan tradition, after death and before one's next birth, when one's consciousness is not connected with a physical body, one experiences a variety of phenomena. These usually follow a particular sequence of degeneration from just after death, the clearest experiences of reality of which one is spiritually capable, and then proceeding to terrifying hallucinations that arise from the impulses of one's previous unskillful actions. For the prepared and appropriately trained individuals, the Bardo offers a state of great opportunity for liberation, since transcendental insight may arise with the direct experience of reality; for others, it can become a place of danger, as the karmically created hallucinations can impel one into a less than desirable rebirth.[21]

Symbolically, Bardo describes times when our usual way of life becomes suspended, as, for example, during a period of illness or during a meditation retreat. Such times can prove fruitful for spiritual progress because external constraints diminish. However, they can also present challenges because our less skillful impulses may come to the foreground, just as in the sidpa Bardo.

The concept of antarabhava,[22] an intervening state between death and rebirth, was brought into Buddhism from the Vedic-Upanishadic philosophical tradition, which later developed into Hinduism.

From the records of ancient Buddhist schools, at least six different groups accepted the notion of an intermediate existence: antarabhava the Sarvastivada, Darstantika, Vatsiputriyas, Sammitiya, Purvasaila and late Mahisasaka. The first four are closely related schools. Opposing them was the Mahasamghika, early Mahisasaka, Theravada, Vibhajyavada and the Sariputra Abhidharma.

To the shaman, the world has three parts: the sky and heavens, earth, and the lower regions or realms.

Each has its own distinctive spirits, many of which influence the world of humans, including souls in crossing over. The upper gods (steng lha) live in the atmosphere and sky. In the middle realm tsen (bar btsan) inhabit the earth, in the lower realm is the home of yoklu (g.yog klu), most notably snake-bodied beings called lu (klu Naga), which live at the bottom of lakes, rivers, and wells and are reported to hoard vast stores of treasure. As all things have a spirit, the spirit living in rocks and trees is called nyen (gnyan); they are often malicious, and Tibetans associate them with sickness and death.

Lu is believed to bring leprosy, and so it is important to keep them away from human habitations. Sadak (sa bdag, "lords of the earth") are beings that live under the ground and are connected with

---

[20] University of California Press eBook Collection, TheSpiritualQuest, (1982 - 2004).
[21] Wikipedia, Bardo.
[22] https://www.wisdomlib.org, Antarabhava,AntarāBhavaDefinitions.

agriculture. Tsen are spirits that live in the atmosphere, and are believed to shoot arrows at humans who disturb them. These cause illness and death. Tsen appears as demonic figures with red skin, wearing helmets and riding over the mountains on red horses. Du (bdud, mara) were apparently originally atmospheric spirits, but they came to be associated with the Buddhist demons called mara, which are led by their king (also named Mara), whose primary goal is to lead sentient beings into ignorance, thus perpetuating the vicious cycle of samsara.

After death, the shaman undertakes a journey to the intermediate world and with the help of their helping spirits seek the soul of the deceased and guide and encourage it to cross over fully, especially if the wandering soul has been affecting the lives of living relatives or otherwise causing problems. Or has been interacting with the spirits in the intermediate realm. During the ritual, blocked energies are released, transformed, and healed so that the soul can receive higher spiritual knowledge when they actually make the crossing.

The shaman may also be asked to help souls and spirits cross over who had no connection to the living. The soul has not crossed over and connected themselves to a living person. That connection causes illness. Usually, the sick individual or their family members will ask a shaman to carry out a divination ceremony where the shaman will determine what is causing the illness. The next step is to act on the reason that has been uncovered. If it is a spirit that has connected themselves to the living, the shaman will perform another ceremony to help it cross over.

The shaman may undertake spiritual battles, confront evil or dark spirits and souls in order to help a sick individual or to help the spirt affecting them to cross over. The upper, middle, and lower realms are also inhabited by the spirits of ancestors [of the sick person] and the shaman must understand them, and may persuade them to help a soul in its current physical incarnation.

The antagonism that often exists between scientifically trained those professing particular religions, there is often little study of each other's accounts of religious and psychic phenomena, so books like those mentioned are often not known outside a narrow circle of experts or academic authorities. Yet Carol Zaleski's[23] book has already spawned a whole academic field of research into the phenomenology of "otherworldly realities"—there have been several international conferences to date—while Sogyal's[24] book is now used worldwide to help people who are nearing death prepare for their passing over. [25]

In Buddhism, some of the earliest references we have to the "intermediate existence" are found in the Sarvastivadin text the Mahavibhasa. For instance, the Mahavibhasa shows a "basic existence," an "intermediate existence," a "birth existence" and "death existence."

The intermediate being who makes the passage in this way from one existence to the next is formed, like every living being, of the five aggregate skandhas[26]. Existence is shown because it cannot have any discontinuity in time and space between the place and moment of death and those of rebirth, and therefore it must be that the two existences belonging to the same series are linked in time and space by an intermediate stage. The intermediate being is the Gandharva, which is as necessary for conception as the fecundity and union of the parents. The Antaraparinirvayin is an Anagamin who gets parinirvana during the intermediary existence. As for the heinous criminal

[23] Wikipedia, CarolZaleski.
[24] SogyalRinpoche.
[25] Dr. Roger J. Woolger, BeyondDeath-TransitionandtheAfterlife.
[26] Wikipedia, Skandha.

guilty of one of the five crimes without interval (Anantara), he passes in quite the same way by an intermediate existence at the end of which he is reborn, necessarily in hell.[27]

What is an intermediate being and an intermediate existence? Intermediate existence, which inserts itself between existence at death and existence at birth, not having arrived at the location where it should go, cannot be said to be born. Between death, the five skandhas of the moment of death—and arising, the five skandhas of the moment of rebirth—there is found an existence—a "body" of five skandhas—that goes to the place of rebirth. This existence between two realms of rebirth (gati) is called an intermediate existence. The skandhas are referred to as heaps because they're merely collections of parts with no central core.

Skandha	Description
Form	Your physical body—traditionally, these are listed as the eyes, ears, nose, tongue, body, and mind.
Feeling	The sensations you experience in your body, including all pain and pleasure.
Perception	You have sense organs, and each of them has objects. Put them together—eye and light, nose and smell, etc.—and you have perception.
Mental	All your concepts and thoughts, from the most mundane to the most grandiose.
Consciousness	Simply put, this is your awareness of the previous skandhas.

Figure 1. Skandha and description

6.3   Six Bardo States

These are transitional states within the 49-day period the soul of the deceased is transitioning to their next life, their rebirth. But Bardo refers to that state in which we have lost our old reality and it is no longer available to us.

What makes death and impermanence so painful is our idea of the strict dichotomy between existence and nonexistence. Knowing something beyond that dualism is paramount. At the moment of death, instead of being caught between the ideas of existence and nonexistence, instead of this crisis of having everything that matters to us taken away all at once, something else can open up entirely; we shift our attention to the nucleus of being, to present itself and experiencing itself.[28]

What makes death and impermanence so painful is our idea of the strict dichotomy between existence and nonexistence. Knowing something beyond that dualism is paramount. At the moment of death, instead of being caught between the ideas of existence and nonexistence, instead of this crisis of having everything that matters to us taken away all at once, something else can open up entirely; we shift our attention to the nucleus of being, to present itself and experiencing itself.[29]

Without some way of managing this experience, this unsettling discontinuity punctuated by occasional disruptions to the very idea of our being, we never know if we are going to show up in

---

[27] Bardo.
[28] Lionsroar.com, TheFourPointsofLettingGointheBardo.
[29] Ibid.

the next moment as a Buddha or as a demon. We're like gods one moment, tasting the fruit of the kingdom, and hungry ghosts the next, not even able to swallow it. How confusing—and how fantastic! This confusion is the raw material of wisdom. Our path is to find a presence in each of these experiences. In the Bardo case, when presence is the only real thing left, if we are searching for security instead, wisdom can be elusive. It's no wonder that religion becomes so poignant during times of crisis; suddenly, presence is all we are. Everything else recedes except what is right in front of us. Recognizing this opens up the potential to experience life with awareness of impermanence and the presence it illuminates.[30]

- Rupture: There is a total rupture in our who-I-am-ness, and we are forced to undergo a great and difficult transformation.

This is the Vajrayana awareness of successive deaths and rebirths, and it is the first essential point to understand: rupture. The more we learn to recognize this sense of disruption, the more willing and able we will be to let go of this notion of an inherent reality and allow that precious pot to slip out of our hands. Rupture takes place all the time, day to day and moment to moment; in fact, as soon as we see our life in terms of these successive deaths and rebirths, we dissolve the very idea of a solid self-grasping onto an inherently real life. We start to see how conditional who-I-am-ness really is and how even that does not provide a reliable ground upon which to stand.

- Emptying the Contrived Self:

This is shunyata[31], which gets translated in various ways, most commonly as "emptiness," but there is no real correlation in our language, no single word or idea that can cover this ground of disrupted reality. Because "emptiness" in English has negative connotations, shunyata is sometimes translated as "voidness," "open spaciousness," and even "boundlessness"; Nyingmas[32] such as Longchenpa explained emptiness in positive terms inextricably associated with presence, clarity, and compassion. But in death and birth, shunyata refers to a direct experience of disruption felt at the core of our being when there is no longer any use manufacturing artificial security.[33]

- Recognize that our experience is based on dynamic, responsive presence.

Our goal is to learn to relax and how to do so and to fall into the inherent peacefulness of not knowing what comes next. When we do—and if we do—everything changes. We are no longer slaves to primordial anxiety.

Experiencing a loss can be freeing. When we are free of all our psychological heaviness and the accumulated weight of our usual momentum, we know the raw presence that remains. To be a Buddhist is to dedicate our lives to abiding in that impermanent, empty, visceral presence. We can bear with greater ease those losses that we know we will inevitably face because we identify with the thread of wakefulness that we meet in all of them. And then perhaps, when death draws near, we can relax with ease into the ground of being as we shed this skin, finally let go of this body, and experience liberation—undefended being in groundless space.[34]

---

[30] Ibid.
[31] www.rigpawiki.org, Emptiness.
[32] NyingmaBuddhism.
[33] Lionsroar.com, TheFourPointsofLettingGointheBardo.
[34] Ibid.

Please See—Bardo, Wikipedia—https://en.wikipedia.org/wiki/Bardo

1. Kyenay Bardo—Skye gnas bar does is the first Bardo of birth and life. This Bardo begins from conception until the last breath when the mind stream withdraws from the body.

2. Milam Bardo—rmi lam bar do is the second Bardo of the dream state. The Milam Bardo is a subset of the first Bardo. Dream Yoga develops practices to integrate the dream state into Buddhist sadhana.

3. Samten Bardo—bsam gtan bar does is the third Bardo of meditation. This Bardo is only experienced by meditators, though individuals may have spontaneous experience of it. Samten Bardo is a subset of the Shinay Bardo.

4. Chikhai Bardo—'chi kha'i bar does is the fourth Bardo of the moment of death. According to tradition, this Bardo is held to begin when the outer and inner signs presage that the onset of death is nigh, and continue through the dissolution or transmutation of the Mahabhuta until the external and internal breath has completed.

   This is the first of three intermediate states between lives in the Tibetan Book of the dead.

5. Chonyid Bardo—chos nyid bar do is the fifth Bardo of the luminosity of true nature, which begins after the final "inner breath" Sanskrit: prana, Vayu; Tibetan: rlung. It is within this Bardo that visions and auditory phenomena occur. In the Dzogchen teachings, these are known as the spontaneously manifesting Thodgal Tibetan: thod-rgyal visions.

   Concomitant to these visions, there is a welling of profound peace and pristine awareness. Sentient beings who have not practised during their lived experience and/or who do not recognize the clear light Tibetan: OD gsal at the moment of death is usually deluded throughout the fifth Bardo of luminosity.

   This is the second of three intermediate states between lives in the Tibetan Book of the dead.

6. Sidpa Bardo—srid pa bar do is the sixth Bardo of becoming or transmigration. This Bardo endures until the inner-breath begins in the new transmigrating form determined by the "karmic seeds" within the storehouse consciousness.

   This is the third of three intermediate states between lives in the Tibetan Book of the dead.

6.4   Bardo Thodol recognizes additional states

C. G. Jung's[35] psychological commentary on the Tibetan Book of the Dead first appeared in an English translation by R. F. C. Hull in the third revised and expanded Evans-Wentz edition of The Tibetan Book of the Dead. The commentary also appears in the Collected Works. Jung applied his

---

[35] Wikipedia, CarlJung.

extensive knowledge of eastern religion to craft a commentary specifically aimed at a western audience unfamiliar with eastern religious tradition and Tibetan Buddhism specifically.[36]

He does not attempt to directly correlate the content of the Bardo Thodol with rituals or dogma found in occidental religion, but highlights karmic phenomena described on the Bardo plane and shows how they parallel unconscious contents both personal and collective encountered in the west, particularly in analytical psychology. [37]

Jung's comments should be taken strictly within the realm of psychology, and not that of theology or metaphysics. Indeed, he repeatedly warns of the dangers for western man in the wholesale adoption of eastern religious traditions, such as yoga. [38]

Bardo Thodol—Tibetan Book of the Dead recognizes three other states.[39]

7. "Life," or ordinary waking consciousness;

8. "Dhyana" (meditation);

   In the oldest texts of Buddhism, dhyāna (Sanskrit) or jhāna (Pali) is the training of the mind, commonly translated as meditation, to withdraw the mind from the automatic responses to sense impressions, leading to a "state of perfect equanimity and awareness (upekkhā-sati-parisuddhi)." Dhyana may have been the core practice of pre-sectarian Buddhism, in combination with several related practices, which together lead to perfected mindfulness and detachment, and are fully realized with the practice of dhyana.

9. "Dream," the dream state during normal sleep.

---

[36] BardoThodol.
[37] Ibid.
[38] Ibid.
[39] Ibid.

What is a Soul?

6.5   Etymology

I n Modern English, the word "soul" is derived from Old English sáwol, sáwel, was first attested in the 8th century poem Beowulf v. 2820 and in the Vespasian Psalter 77.50. It is cognate with other German and Baltic terms for the same idea, including Gothic saiwala, Old High German sêula, sêla, Old Saxon sêola, Old Low Franconian sêla, sîla, Old Norse sála, and Lithuanian siela. Deeper etymology of the Germanic word is unclear.[40]

The original concept behind the Germanic root is thought to mean "coming from or belonging to the sea (or lake)," because of the Germanic and pre-Celtic belief in souls emerging from and returning to sacred lakes, Old Saxon sêola (soul) compared to Old Saxon sêo (sea).[41]

6.6   A Definition

The word "soul" can refer to the Spirit of God. Or, if the person speaking to me does not want to refer to "God," just "Spirit." It exists in each individual; it is an ever-existing, ever-conscious, ever-new bliss.

Identification of Soul with the physical body, and becomes the nature of the individual. References to "spiritual progress" or "soul evolution" use this definition, because the soul that is aware of its true identity as part of God is already perfect. Souls only develop or progress in the sense that they go from identifying with their physical bodies to identifying with God. This can also be called the ego.

6.7   Dictionary Definition

Merriam-Webster Dictionary[42]

- the immaterial essence, animating principle, or actuating cause of an individual life

- the spiritual principle embodied in human beings, all rational and spiritual beings, or the universe

- Capitalized, Christian Science: GOD senses

- a person's total self

- an active or essential part

- of a moving spirit: LEADER

Figure 2. The Soul

---

40 Wikipedia, Soul.
41 Ibid.
42 Merriam-Webster Dictionary, DefinitionofSoulbyMerriam-Webster.

- the moral and emotional nature of human beings

- the quality that arouses emotion and sentiment

- spiritual or moral force: FERVOUR

6.8   Atman–Hinduism

Atman is a Sanskrit word that means inner self, spirit, or soul. In Hindu philosophy, especially in the Vedanta school of Hinduism, Atman is the first principle: the true self of an individual beyond identification with phenomena, the essence of an individual. In order to attain liberation (moksha), a human being must gain self-knowledge, which is to realize that one's true self is identical with the transcendent self-Brahman.

The six orthodox schools of Hinduism believe that there is Atman (soul, self) in every being. This is a major point of difference with the Buddhist doctrine of Anatta, which holds that there is no unchanging soul or self.

6.9   Theological Soul

Soul and the spirit are the two primary immaterial parts that Scripture ascribes to humanity.43 The word spirit refers only to the immaterial facet of humanity. Human beings have a spirit, but we are not spirits. However, the words soul and spirit are often used interchangeably; the primary distinction between soul and spirit is that in men and women the soul has animated life, or is the seat of the senses, desires, affections, and appetites.

The soul, in many religious, philosophical, and mythological traditions, is the ethereal essence of a living being. The soul or psyche comprises the mental abilities of a living being: reason, character, feeling, consciousness, memory, perception, thinking, etc. Depending on the philosophical system, a soul can either be mortal or immortal.44 The soul is alive, physically and eternally. The spirit can be alive, as with believers (1 Peter 3:18), or dead as unbelievers are (Colossians 2:13; Ephesians 2:4-5).

Believers in Jesus Christ and his role in salvation respond to the things that come from the Spirit of God, understanding and discerning them spiritually. The spirit allows us to connect, or not, with God. Our spirits relate to His Spirit, either accepting his promptings and conviction, proving that we belong to him (Romans 8:16) or resisting him and proving that we do not have a spiritual life (Acts 7:51).

The spirit is the element in humanity that gives us the ability to have an intimate relationship with God. Whenever the word spirit is used, it refers to the immaterial part of humanity that "connects" with God, who himself is spirit (John 4:24).

Judaism and Christianity teach that only human beings have immortal souls, although immortality is disputed within Judaism and the concept of immortality may have been influenced by Plato.

---

43 GotQuestions.org, WhatIstheDifferencebetweentheSoulandSpiritofMan?.
44 Wikipedia, Soul.

The "origin of the soul" has provided a vexing question in Christianity. The major theories put forward include soul creationism, traducianism, and pre-existence. According to soul creationism, God creates each individual soul created directly, either at the moment of conception or some later time. According to traducianism, the soul comes from the parents by natural generation. According to the pre-existence theory, the soul exists before the moment of conception. There have been differing thoughts regarding whether human embryos have souls from conception, or whether there is a point between conception and birth where the fetus gains a soul, consciousness, and/or personhood. Stances in this question might play a role in judgments on the morality of abortion.[45]

The most basic meaning of "soul" is "life." There is no distinction whether it refers to physical or eternal life. Jesus asks what it profits a man to gain the entire world and lose his soul, referring to his eternal life (Matthew 16:26). Both Old and New Testaments reiterate we are to love God completely, with the whole "soul," which refers to everything that is in us that makes us alive (Deuteronomy 6:4-5; Mark 12:30). Whenever the word "soul" is used, it can refer to the whole person, whether physically alive or in the afterlife.

The soul is our source of absolute uniqueness, a place within that connects you not only to your own value and essence, but to the value and essence of every other living being. This is limiting. We will get back to that later.

6.10   Where Is the Soul in the Physical Body?

Debate on "where" the soul is in a physical body is a large and disruptive discussion topic. Mostly because we do not have a suitable definition by which to recognize the soul if we are lucky enough or astute enough to find it!

- Descartes: The pineal gland is a tiny organ in the centre of the brain that played an important role in Descartes's philosophy. He regarded it as the principal seat of the soul and the place in which all our thoughts are formed.[46]

- Leonardo da Vinci used his experience in anatomy to hypothesize that the soul was in the optic chiasm, near the third ventricle of the brain. His views were supported by observations of change in perception following disturbances to that area of the brain.[47]

- Aristotle in De Anima (On the Soul) suggests that the organs of the body are required for the soul to interact with. Unlike Plato, Aristotle believed the soul's existence was not separate from the human body; thus, the soul could not be immortal. Similarly, to Plato, however, Aristotle believed the soul is composed of three parts: the vegetative, sensitive, and rational. Growth and reproduction result from the vegetative soul, and are found in all organisms. The sensitive soul, however, allows for sensation and movement in humans and animals. Third, the rational is exclusive to humans, and allows for rational thought.[48]

---

[45] Ibid.
[46] Stanford Encyclopedia of Philosophy, DescartesandthePinealGland.
[47] Wikipeda, HistoryoftheLocationoftheSoul.
[48] Ibid.

6.11 Ensoulment

After considering "where" the soul can be found in the body, how does it get there, when does it arrive?

In religion, ensoulment is the moment at which a human being gains a soul.[49] [50] Some religions say that a soul is newly created within a developing child and others, especially in religions that believe in reincarnation[51], that the soul is pre-existing and added at a particular stage of development. In the time of Aristotle, it was widely believed that the human soul entered the forming body at 40 days (male embryos) or 90 days (female embryos), and quickening showed a soul. Other religious views are that ensoulment happens at the moment of conception; or when the child takes the first breath after being born; at the formation of the nervous system and brain; at the first brain activity (e.g., heartbeat); or when the fetus can survive independently of the uterus (viability).[52]

The concept is closely related to debates on the morality of abortion and the morality of contraception. Religious beliefs that human life has an innate sacredness to it have motivated many statements by spiritual leaders of various traditions over the years. However, the three matters are not exactly parallel, given that various figures have argued that some kind of life without a soul, in various contexts, still has a moral worth that must be considered. [53]

6.12 Shamanic Soul

The Catholic theologian Thomas Aquinas[54]attributed "soul" to all organisms but argued that only human souls are immortal. Other religions, most notably Hinduism and Jainism, hold that all living things, from the smallest bacterium, to the largest mammals, are the souls themselves and have their physical representative, the body, in the world. The actual self is the soul; the body is simply a mechanism to experience the karma of that life. Thus, if we see a tiger, then there is a self-conscious identity or soul living in it, and a physical representative of the whole body of the tiger, which is observable in the world. Some teach that even non-biological entities such as rivers and mountains possess souls. This belief is called animism.[55]

Animism is a major part of the shamanic worldview and an understanding of what this world represents. Shamans often work by being able to reach a different level of consciousness or awareness that allows them to speak to the spirits of the natural world, who can then provide them with knowledge and information. Shamanism often relies pretty heavily on animistic ideas with most shamanistic practices, but not all but animism can exist without shamanism.

Your soul lives inside your body in the physical world, but it also lives in the Soul World at the same time. Everyone and everything are in the Soul World because everyone and everything have a soul.

The soul is the principle of life, feeling, thought, and action in humans. In some religions, it is believed that when the person dies, although their body is no longer alive, their spirit or soul moves

---

[49] Wikipedia, AscendedMaster.
[50] https://en.wikipedia.org/wiki/The_City_of_God, TheCityofGod.
[51] http://healerofheartsandminds.com, Reincarnation,PastLives,SufferingandtheBible,aShaman'sViews.
[52] Wikipedia, AscendedMaster.
[53] Ibid.
[54]
[55] Wikipedia, Soul.

on to another world. The soul in religion is needed for reincarnation, which is clear in Hinduism and Buddhism, where when we die, our souls come back to take over the body of any living matter. Souls are not only clear in religion but also in philosophy.

6.13 Shamanism and Animism

Bon is both a shamanist and an animistic[56]religion.

Shamans have visions and perform various deeds during a trance and it is believed they have the power to control spirits in the body. They may leave normal existence and travel or fly to other worlds. Manchu-Tungus nomads of Siberia and northern Chinese language, Shaman means "agitated or frenzied people."

Shamans are bridges between their communities and the spiritual world. During trances, which are induced during a ritual, shamans seek spirits to help cure illnesses, bring about pleasant weather, predict the future, or communicate with deceased ancestors.

Animism attributes a distinct spiritual essence or soul to plants, inanimate objects, and natural phenomena. It is a belief in a supernatural power that organizes and animates the material universe and that ancestors watch over the living from the spirit world.

There are places on earth where sacred power is concentrated. Those places are held sacred and where communication with the spirit world takes place.

6.14 Bon Sarma

Often referred to as New Bon, this is an eclectic tradition combining elements of Indian Buddhism and Yungdrung Bon, which appeared in the eighth century AD and is still very popular in eastern Tibet, particularly in Kham.[57]

6.15   Mixed Bon

This refers to the wide range of tribal traditions practised in the borderlands surrounding Tibet and the Himalayas, in which Prehistoric Bon, Yungdrung Bon and various other elements mingle in various proportions.[58]

6.16 Bo Murgel

The Bo Murgel belief system of Mongolia and Buryatia—thousands of miles from Tibet—has many features in common with Tibetan Bon, not least of which is its name, Bo—pronounced like "bore" with a double "or" sound. [59]

---

[56] Animism.
[57] Dmitry Ermakov, BoandBon-AncientShamanicTraditionsofSiberiaandTibetinTheirRelationtotheTeachingsofaCentralAsianBuddha.
[58] Ibid.
[59] Ibid.

6.17 Dzogchen?

Dzogchen or "Great Perfection," it is a tradition of teachings in Tibetan Buddhism aimed at discovering and continuing in the natural primordial state of being. It is a central teaching of the Yungdrung-Bon tradition and in the Nyingma school of Tibetan Buddhism. In these traditions, Dzogchen is the highest and most definitive path of the nine vehicles to liberation.[60] According to this terma, Dzogchen originated with the founder of the Bon tradition, Tonpa Shenrab.

6.18 Soul Channels

Open your spiritual channels to be a better parent, spouse, partner, friend, teacher, or healer. When you open your spiritual channels, you access wisdom and guidance to become your best self. Your soul has great wisdom, knowledge, and experience of hundreds or thousands of lifetimes and from your spiritual fathers and mothers in Heaven. Your soul has great love and care for you because your physical journey scars your soul's journey. Your own beloved soul is your best friend and one of your best guides.[61]

Open your spiritual channels to receive guidance and wisdom from your spiritual fathers and mothers in Heaven and from the Divine. Soul Language and Translation Soul Language is the universal language. Every soul can communicate with any other soul through Soul Language. [62]

---

[60] Wikipedia, Dzogchen.
[61] Master Sha Tao Center Honolulu, OpenSpiritualChannelsSoulLanguageandTranslation-HonoluluTaoHealingSoulHealingEnergyHealingMasterSha.
[62] Ibid.

7   Signs of Soul Loss

To a shaman "soul loss," a loss of meaning, direction, vitality, mission, purpose, identity, and genuine connection; a deep unhappiness that, unfortunately, most of us consider as simply ordinary. The soul is our source of absolute uniqueness, a place within that connects you not only to your own value and essence, but to the value and essence of every other living being. What makes soul loss so subtle and dangerous is that very few people have realized that it has happened. Most of us do not know that we have disconnected from our soul and accept as normal a numbness and lack of meaning in our lives. [Lissa Rankin, MD[63]]

Because we all belong to this culture, we all suffer from soul loss. Soul loss is an epidemic and blinds us from seeing the potential for joy and wholeness in ordinary life. When you heal from soul

Figure 4. The Soul

Figure 3. Signs of Soul Loss

---

[63] Lissa Rankin https://lissarankin.com, DiagnosticSignsThatYou'reSufferingfromSoulLoss.

loss, you see familiar things in new ways so you can increase your joy in what you already have.
[Lissa Rankin, MD[64]]

---

[64] Ibid.

Diagnostic Signs that show soul loss: [Lissa Rankin, MD[65]]

#	Description
1	You feel you're not as good as other people.
2	You yearn to be of service, but you do not know what you have to contribute and why it matters.
3	You strive in vain for an impossible-to-achieve standard of perfection.
4	Your fears keep you from living large.
5	You are frequently worried that you're not good enough, smart enough, thin enough, young enough, [fill in the blank] enough.
6	You feel like a victim of circumstances that are beyond your control.
7	You feel like your daily life is meaningless and task-driven.
8	You often feel helpless, hopeless, or pessimistic.
9	You protect your heart with steel walls.
10	You often feel you don't really matter and your love doesn't make a difference.
11	You're always trying to fit in and belong, but you rarely feel you do.
12	You feel beaten down by the challenges you face in your life.
13	You suffer from a variety of vague, hard to treat physical symptoms, such as fatigue, chronic pain, weight gain or loss, insomnia, skin disorders, or gastrointestinal symptoms.
14	You struggle with being able to accept love and nurturing.
15	You feel depressed, anxious, or chronically worried.
16	You feel you're not appreciated enough.
17	You often judge others.
18	You frequently numb yourself with alcohol, drugs, sex, television, or excessive busyness.
19	You feel disappointed with life.
20	You've forgotten how to dream.

---

[65] Ibid.

8   Soul Loss and the Retrieval of the Elemental Energies

In the Tibetan tradition, there is the notion of "soul loss." Although this is an imbalance of the elements, it is greater than the imbalances suffered in normal life. It is a question of degree. Soul loss is a profound loss of elemental qualities and a condition of extreme imbalance that usually, though not always, is caused by traumatic external situations and beings.[66]

We say that the soul can be stolen by malevolent beings of the eight classes, which are described in section Eight Classes of Being in this book.

These negative, non-physical external beings damage our capacity for positive human qualities. This usually happens during trauma, such as emotional or physical abuse, an accident, loss of a loved one, assault, rape, incest, divorce, surgery, or wartime experiences. The soul part leaves as a protective mechanism. In indigenous cultures, the soul part is retrieved by a shaman shortly after the trauma. In our culture, people can go their entire lifetime without the soul part. [67]

Someone may also lose part of their soul by giving it to a loved one through a desire to share themselves with another. Sometimes, a soul part may be stolen. [68]

Psychologically, this phenomenon is understood in terms of dissociation, and it is a brilliant survival mechanism for the human psyche. The major characteristic of all dissociative phenomena involves a detachment from reality, rather than a loss of reality as in psychosis.[69]

What has been lost can be retrieved by the shaman through the practice and rituals of Soul Retrieval. The ritual is complicated and requires instruction and teaching by a qualified master.

The shaman first needs to speak to and understand the recipient of the soul retrieval. He or she needs to understand what is missing, what has been damaged, so that they may undertake the soul retrieval ritual. Some will call this a diagnosis.

During the ritual, the shaman will enter an altered state of consciousness, or ASC. This may be achieved by dance, rhythmic drumming, plant-based hallucinogens, or alcohol. However, not all shamans use these techniques; each shaman is unique and uses different techniques to reach the state they need to soul journey.

During the soul journey, the Shaman will join with either a main helping spirit or a series of spirits that will aid in the search for the soul, which may be more fragmented. At this point in the ritual, the shaman and helping spirts must determine the state of the soul and/or its fragments and what healing needs to be undertaken before it is given back to the recipient. It also needs to be determined if the souls or fragments are being held hostage by a spirit and what the intention of that spirit is.

The shaman negotiates with the hostage taker in order to get back the soul or piece they are holding on to. A special, separate ritual may have to be completed in order to satisfy the hostage

---

[66] Tenzin Wangyal Rinpoche, SoulRetrievalandRelatedIdeas.

[67] Theinnervoyage.com, SoulRetrieval.

[68] Ibid.

[69] Wikipedia, DissociationPsychology.

taker. In some situations, a struggle may be undertaken by the shaman and they're helping spirits and the hostage taker to pull back the soul or otherwise free the soul.

In all the activity of searching and possibly struggling with a spirit, the shaman must protect his or her own spirit. Ensure it remains intact and is not damaged by the actions undertaken. The strength of the helping spirits and experience of the shaman in preforming soul retrieval is essential to the success of the ritual.

Once the shaman and their helping spirits have gathered the soul and any fragments and have healed them, they must be returned to the recipient. The traditional reintegration of the soul with the recipient's physical being is through breath. The shaman breathes hard at or on the recipient and matches the intensity, intending to send the soul back to them, and focusing on returning their light. The soul or soul fragments at this stage are like lost children being returned to their parents.

Then we support the client to integrate this extra energy, at first just allowing the energy to sink down into their bones and cells, which goes deeply into the recipient.

8.1   Element Retrieval

As with soul retrieval, the elemental energy of a recipient may be lost, stolen, or so seriously unbalanced, it may appear that a particular element is being taken away.

Sutra, Tantra, and the shamanic vehicles include practices to reconnect us to the positive qualities. This process is not just about having pleasant experiences; it is about connecting to deeper aspects of ourselves. Although ultimately, we need to go beyond the simplicity of positive and negative, until we actually do, positive qualities lead us closer to the experience of the base of existence, while negative qualities distract us and lead further into abstraction.[70]

When elemental qualities are lost, there is a flattening of experience, a loss of richness and resonance. This is like the experience of a broken heart. A man or woman loses a spouse or partner shockingly, is betrayed or abandoned, and he or she closes the heart. This is a familiar theme in novels and movies: the person can't love because of the fear of being hurt again. The same inner damage can happen when someone loses a child, is raped, witness's brutality, is subjected to brutality, goes through a war, is in a car accident, or loses a house—the catastrophes and calamities that fall upon us humans. The shock to the soul overwhelms it with fear, loss, or some other powerful emotion and, and the result is the loss of positive qualities, losing life force and vitality, losing joy and empathy. It may also result in physical frailty and losing sensory clarity.[71]

Regardless of whether losing elemental energy is sudden or occurs over time, or results from a traumatizing or dehumanizing environment, the damage to the energy of the elements and their balance in the recipient occurs. The cause is a negative spirit or spirits.

When we are physically weakened, our physical body is susceptible to bacterial and virus infections from bacteria and viruses. When we are psychically weakened, we are susceptible to the influences of negative non-physical beings.

---

[70] Tenzin Wangyal Rinpoche, TibetanSoulRetrieval.
[71] SoulRetrievalandRelatedIdeas.

After an accident, for instance, an individual may experience lethargy, a loss of inspiration and creativity, or a loss of vigour. This condition may heal naturally, but if it doesn't, if fire element energy has been lost, it can become chronic. This may show up in work and in relationships, and may manifest in the body as an illness and in the mind as a disturbance in cognitive activity. The accident is the apparent physical cause of the loss, but the actual loss is caused by trauma or can come as the person is weakened and vulnerable to malevolent external beings. In either case, the damage is manifested in the soul.[72]

Element retrieval also refers to the overabundance of an element which causes spiritual imbalance. The shaman must soul journey to discover the source of the abundance and remove it, and, after removing it, the shaman must rebalance the elements and manage any damage by the time there was the overabundance of the element. If someone is too grounded because of the imbalance, the shaman must support the elements of Air and Space, for example.

---

[72] Ibid.

8.2   Blocked or Closed Chakras.

The Chakras are the central energy system of the body in which the soul and spirit are travelling. They are the energy conduit from the root to the crown. If you look at the function of each chakra, and the dependence of the physical body and spirit on each, it is apparent that blockage or restriction will limit not just the body but the spirit and soul.

Depending on the impact to us by events such as being betrayed by a lover, the loss of a loved one or a parent and a physical accident, one or more of our chakras may have become blocked or restricted. If you sit quietly, eyes closed, warm, comfortable and breathing normally. No external distractions. Clear your mind, let all distracting thoughts pass. Feel your quietness.

Rituals to unblock or remove restrictions in a recipient's chakras may be carried out to return the strength and vibrancy of the chakras affected. This also requires the shaman to engage in balancing and ensuring a clear flow of energy from the root to the crown chakra.

8.3   The Root Chakra

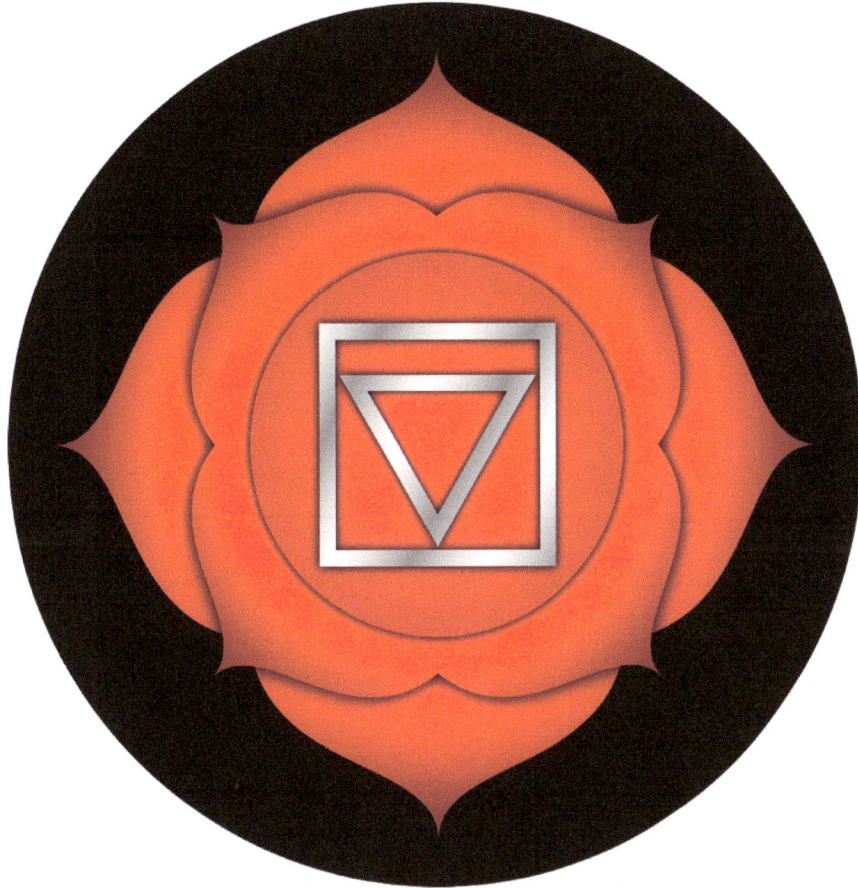

Figure 5. Root Chakra. Image by Peter Lomas from Pixabay

Colour—red

Element—Earth

Seed Sound—LANG

Location—At the base of the spine, where the tail bone is located

Sanskrit—Muladhara—translation root or base support

Physical anatomy engaged—sacrum, coccygeal nerve plexus, adrenal glands, feet, legs, hips, bones, large intestines, anus, and skin.

A healthy Root chakra is reflected in one feeling grounded, connected to the earth, comfortable in their body and present in physical surroundings. They feel responsible and well able to ensure their own safety and security and their family in the physical world, emotionally and spiritually. Boundaries, setting them and adhering to them are important for this chakra. A balanced Root Chakra supports a prosperous lifestyle.—as we live in a material world, this can be helpful for generating income, paying bills on time, saving for the future and easing the stress that comes with an inability to do so.

Proper functioning of the Root Chakra fosters proper energy flow throughout the body, giving the chakra system a firm foundation on which the other energy centres may function. The Chakra represents a sense of security, safety, ability to survive, groundedness, your place in the world, financial state and physical health.

If your Root Chakra is blocked, you may feel threatened, panicked, or anxious. Insecure, fearful, lack of personal boundaries, flightiness, anxiety, disorganization, financial problems, eating disorders, constipation, and problems with the feet, legs, hips, and bones

This anxiety can easily infiltrate your thoughts, making everything suddenly feel uncertain. You may also find that you can't concentrate and that you're constantly preoccupied with worries about your well-being. In some people, this can manifest as hypochondria or general paranoia. Physical issues potentially caused by a blocked Root Chakra include a sore lower back, low energy levels, and cold extremities.

Overloaded symptoms are hoarding, greed, materialism, obesity, overly strict boundaries, obsession with body balance by eating protein and root vegetables, sleeping more, massage, exercise and feeling your feet against the earth.

If your Root Chakra is blocked, you may feel threatened, panicked, or anxious. This anxiety can easily infiltrate your thoughts, making everything suddenly feel uncertain. You may also find that you can't concentrate and that you're constantly preoccupied with worries about your well-being. In some people, this can manifest as hypochondria or general paranoia. Physical issues potentially caused by a blocked Root Chakra include a sore lower back, low energy levels, and cold extremities.

Yoga poses that will help balance this chakra—Apanasana, Supported Malasana, Supported Malasana Twists, Salabhasana, Setu Bandha Sarvangasana, Janu Sirsasana, Mountain, Trees, and Corpse pose.

8.4   The Sacral Chakra

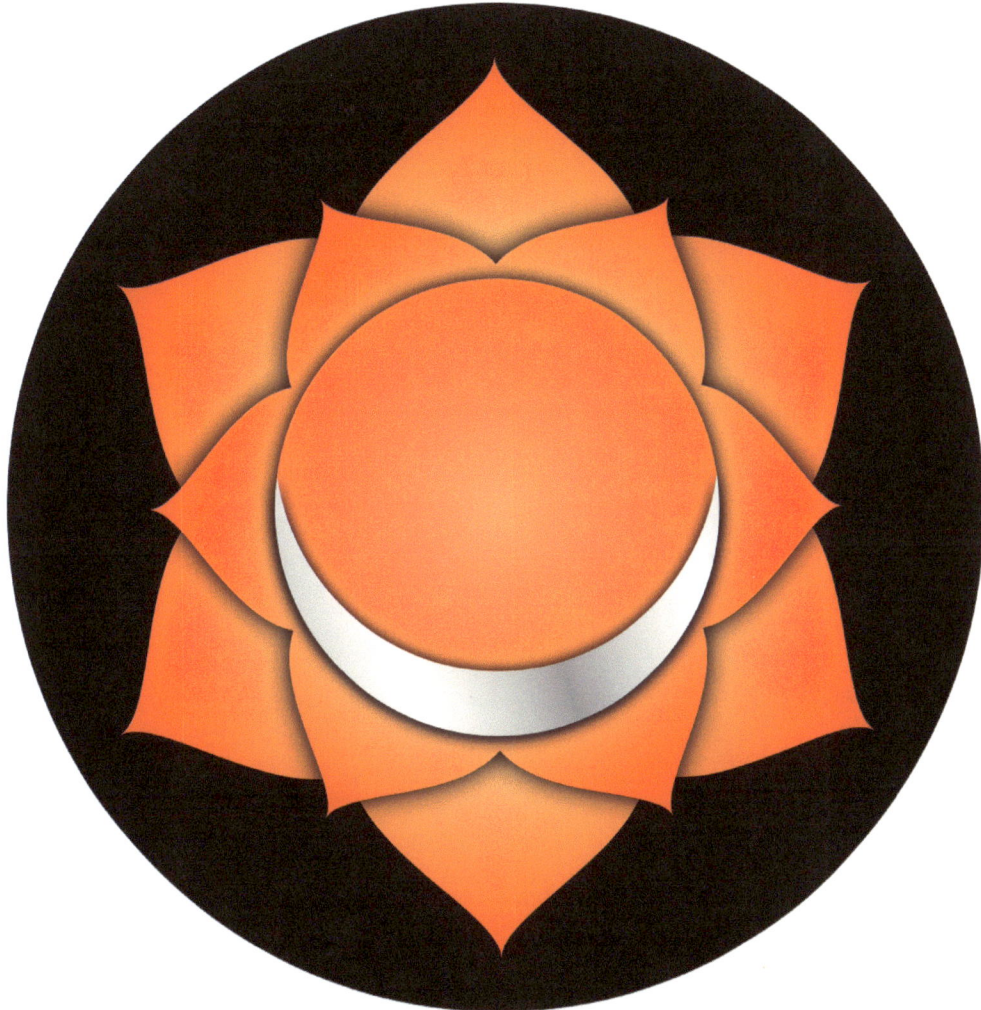

Figure 6. Sacral Chakra Image by Peter Lomas from Pixabay

Colour—Orange

Element—water

Seed sound—VANG

Location—just below the belly button

Sanskrit—Svadhisthana—translation—dwelling of the Self

Physical anatomy engaged—Abdomen, sacral nerve plexus, genitals, reproductive organs, kidneys, and bladder

This Chakra is the source of all of your creativity, your sexuality and your relationships. Unlike the roundedness of the Root Chakra, this chakra is free flowing and fluid. The Chakra is one step removed from any preoccupations about survival and safety, and represents the instinctual sensory perception of the world.

Balancing this chakra means you can allow yourself to FEEL emotion without BEING the emotion. Recognizing emotions as pleasurable or painful, whether mellow or deeply intense, as simply feelings that enhance and are a part of our human journey without the belief that WE ARE that emotion—we are always ourselves and the emotion is merely a feeling to be experienced—this is a balanced Sacral Chakra.

An excellent indicator of whether a person's sacral chakra is balanced can be gained by the way they 'move.' Do they move gracefully and confidently without awkwardness or clumsiness? Do they stomp or float around?

Attempting to move more purposefully and gracefully will aid in balancing this chakra.

When there's a problem with the Sacral Chakra, you're likely to feel bored, listless and uninspired. You may have a low sex drive, and you'll possibly feel afraid of (or resistant to) change. Physical symptoms associated with a blocked Sacral Chakra can include urinary discomfort, increased allergies, and an attraction to addictive behaviours. These need not be related to drug or alcohol use. Shopping addiction, gambling, and issues with eating can all be linked to issues with the Sacral Chakra.

Blocked symptoms are creative blocks, infertility, sexual problems, stiffness, problems with intimate relationships, an inability to feel pleasure and resistance to change. Urinary discomfort, increased allergies, and an attraction to addictive behaviours. These need not be related to drug or alcohol use. Shopping addiction, gambling, and issues with eating can all be linked to issues with the Sacral Chakra.

Overloaded symptoms are over-emotionality, addictions, obsession with sex, hyper-flexibility, PMS, and excessive dependence on others

Balancing suggestions include getting professional help for addictions and relationship problems, pursuing creativity, swimming, ballet, and spending time with immediate family.

Yoga poses help balance this chakra—Dwipada Pitham, Salamba Bhujangasana, Jathara Parivrtti, Kapotasana, Supta Baddha Konasana, Dhanurasana, Sun Salutation

8.5   The Solar Plexus Chakra

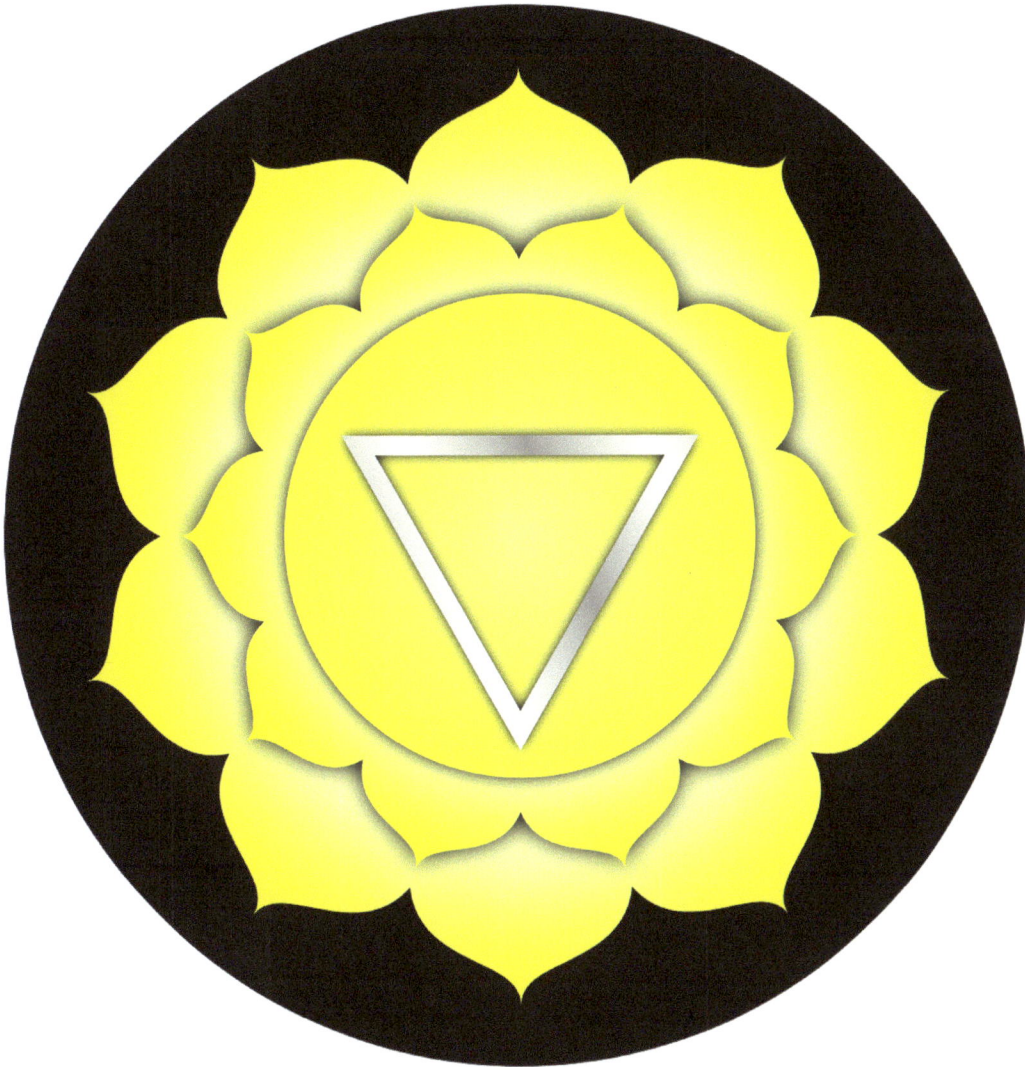

Figure 7. Solar Plexus Chakra. Image by Peter Lomas from Pixabay

Colour—Yellow

Element—fire

Seed sound—RANG

Location—just below the rib cage

Sanskrit—Manipura—translation—dwelling place of the jewel
Physical anatomy engaged—Solar plexus, stomach, digestive organs, upper intestines, middle back, liver, pancreas, gallbladder, muscles

This Solar Plexus chakra is where you open to all abundance, prosperity, and opportunities. Imagine a beam of yellow light pouring through this chakra when you need to give your confidence a boost. This chakra focuses on who you are, what you can do and how you can do it.

Understanding and accepting who you are giving you a strong sense of self and an ability to get things done.

Represents a sense of self, ego, self-esteem, willpower, and ability to get things done

Blocked symptoms are low self-esteem, sluggishness, victim mentality, low energy, chronic fatigue, weak core muscles, slow digestion, poor appetite and problems with pancreas, gallbladder, and liver. Confidence will be very shaky. If there is only a small blockage, there may only be insecurity in one specific area. A larger blockage will cause generalized self-esteem problems. You might be haunted by thoughts that you are not good enough. Or you may feel unable to draw useful lessons from life's challenges. Physical difficulties associated with a blocked Solar Plexus Chakra may include digestive discomfort and troubles with memory.

Overloaded symptoms are aggressiveness, arrogance, too much energy, irritability, violence, ambitiousness at the expense of others, an inability to feel empathy, high stress, hypertension, muscle spasms and overuse of painkillers or sedatives.

Balancing suggestions include working up a sweat, doing hot yoga, sitting in a sauna or steam room, spending time in the sun, listening to others, slowing down and strengthening muscles in your core.

Yoga poses for balancing this chakra—Tadasana, Virabhadrasana I, Dhanurasana, Surya Namaskar and Navasana.

8.6   The Heart Chakra

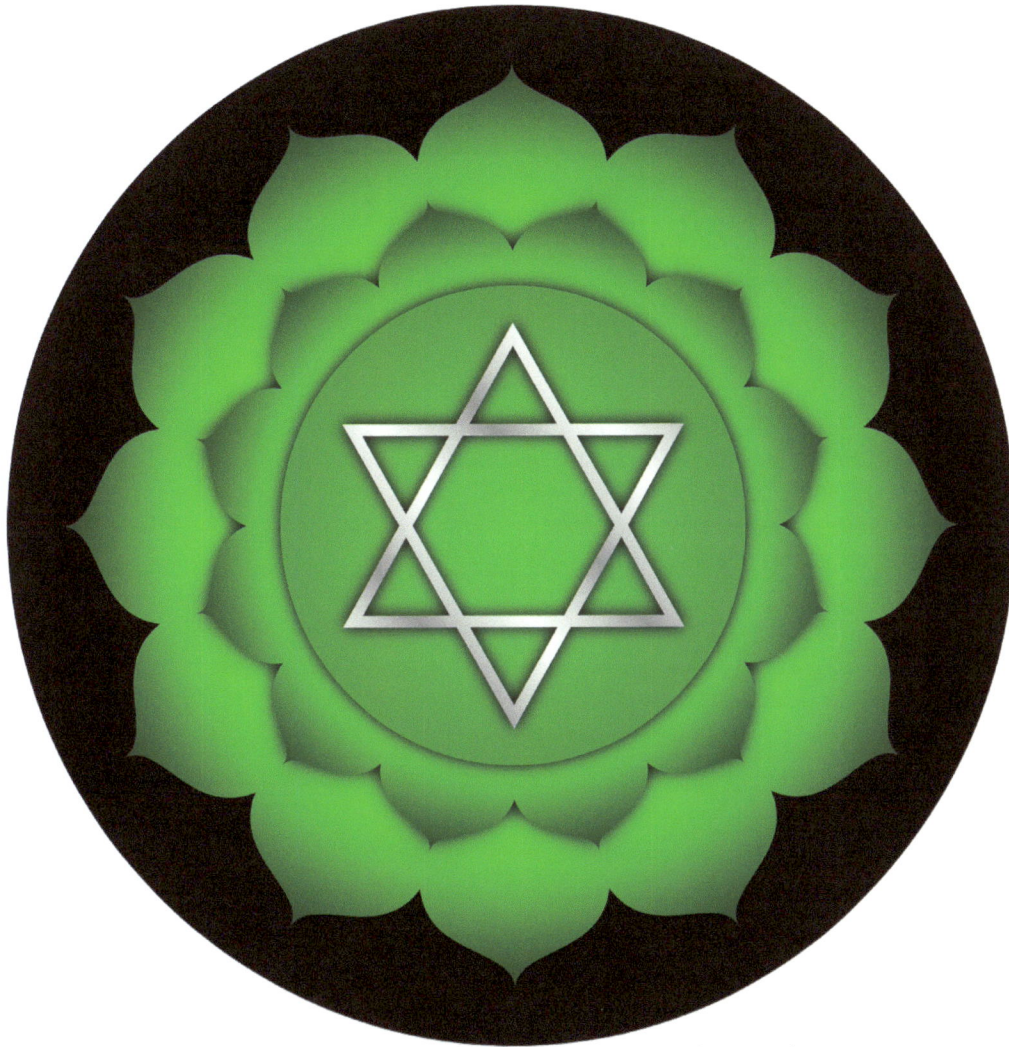

Figure 8. Heart Chakra. Image by Peter Lomas from Pixabay

Colour—Green

Element—Air

Seed Sound—YANG

Location—behind the heart

Sanskrit—Anahata translation—sunstruck or intact "The heart sings without being played." Physical anatomy engaged—heart, lungs, shoulders, arms, chest, breasts, thymus gland, cardiac nerve plexus.

This chakra is the "connector chakra" between earthly and spiritual chakras. The balance and strength and compassion that you find within your Heart Chakra will be reflected in all areas of your life and in everything that you do. A healthy and open-Heart Chakra enhances your healing ability when used on Self or others. Improving your posture automatically opens your Heart Chakra more fully.

The Chakra represents your ability to give and receive love, your capacity to love yourself and your sense of compassion and empathy for all beings.

Blocked symptoms include heart disease, lung problems, relationship problems, commitment issues, fear of intimacy, being judgmental and an inability to feel compassion, and you'll struggle to relate to other people. You will be less compassionate than usual and may be impatient. You'll commonly find it harder than usual to trust, and you won't feel at peace. Rather, you'll feel restless and disgruntled. A blocked Heart Chakra can also manifest physically. Some Chakra experts think such a misalignment may be linked to issues like high blood pressure and low immune system function.

Overloaded symptoms include chest pain, breast problems, including cancer, self-sacrificing behaviour, codependency and ignoring your own needs in the constant service of other balancing suggestions include taking care of yourself, practising breathing exercises, doing yoga that opens the chest (back bends) or nurtures the heart. Childs pose and by loving in better balance, giving and receiving love without sacrificing yourself or taking energy from your other Chakras.

Yoga poses to aid in balancing this chakra—Bhujangasana, Gomukhasana, Garudasana, Ustrasana, Matsyasana, Marjaryasana, Urdhva Mukha Svanasana,

8.7   The Throat Chakra

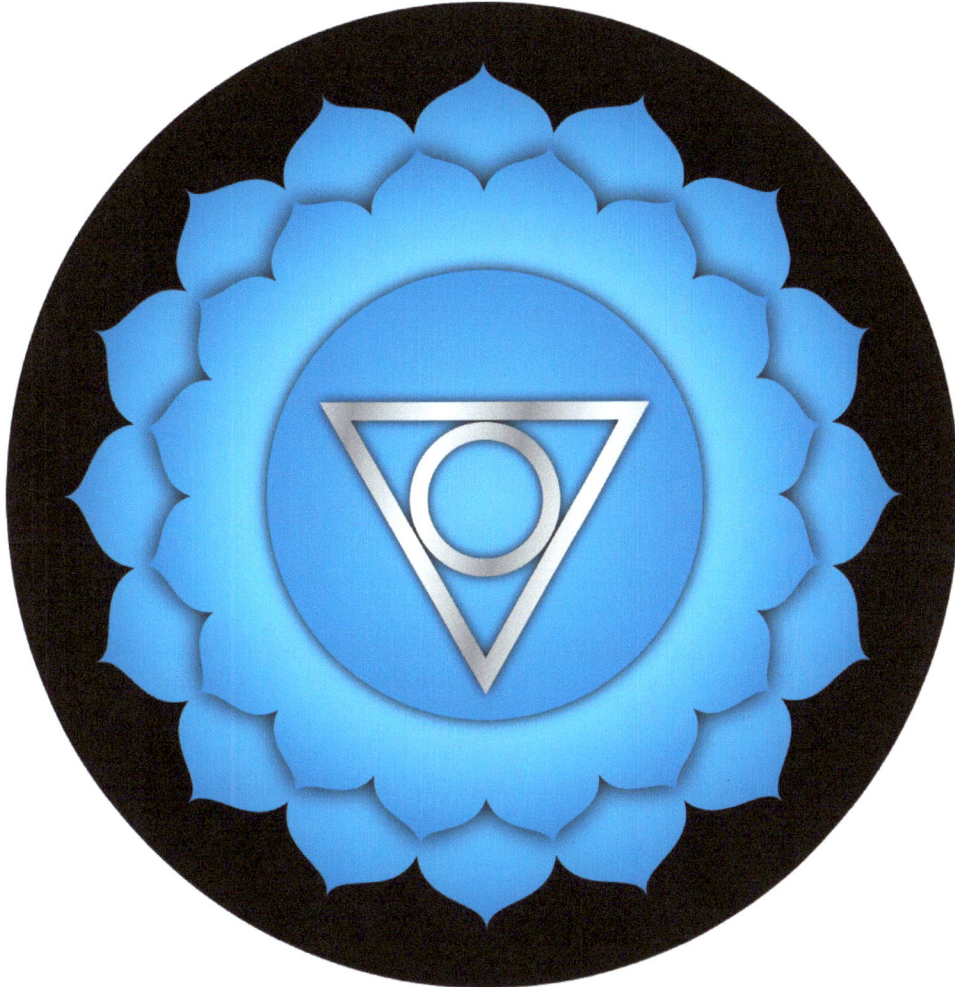

Figure 9. Throat Chakra. Image by Peter Lomas from Pixabay

Colour—Sky Blue

Element—Sound

Seed Sound—HANG

Location—in the throat

Sanskrit—Vishuddha translation—purity

Physical anatomy engaged—throat, trachea, esophagus, neck, thyroid gland, cervical spine, mouth, jaw, teeth

This chakra is the centre for communication, sound, vibration, and TRUTH. Simple expression through vocal expression, drawing, writing and/or musical ability and good listening abilities are all part of this balanced chakra. Speaking your truth, hearing and UNDERSTANDING the truth in what others are saying are continued strengths here. Honouring the vibration and rhythm of your voice [spoken voice, written voice, musical voice] aids in the healthy balance of your Throat chakra.

Represents your ability to communicate, express yourself, listen, speak truth, hear the truth, and understand the meaning behind and beyond words.

Blocked symptoms include a weak voice, laryngitis, throat pain, neck pain, stiff neck, jaw pain, hypothyroidism, dental problems, writer's block, lack of musical ability and problems expressing yourself. There is an inability to say what you really want to say. You may feel you're stuck holding onto secrets. Similarly, you may believe that people don't want to hear your thoughts, or that you can't find the right words for your feelings.

Once again, a small blockage may mean you only struggle with self-expression at work, or with a particular friend. Meanwhile, a significant misalignment may mean you constantly feel thwarted in communication. Physically, a blocked Throat Chakra may present with pain in the neck, sensitivity to hormone fluctuations, and discomfort in throat tissue.

Overloaded symptoms include neck problems, hyperthyroidism/talking too much/talking too loudly, interrupting, and speaking without regard for other people's feelings.

Balancing suggestions include singing, humming, listening to music, writing, talking to people, listening to people, practising silence and getting a shoulder and neck massage.

Yoga poses to assist with balancing this chakra—Start with an easy neck release, Bhujangasana, Matsyasana, Salamba Sarvangasana, Viparita Kirani and Jalandhara Bandha.

8.8   The Third Eye Chakra

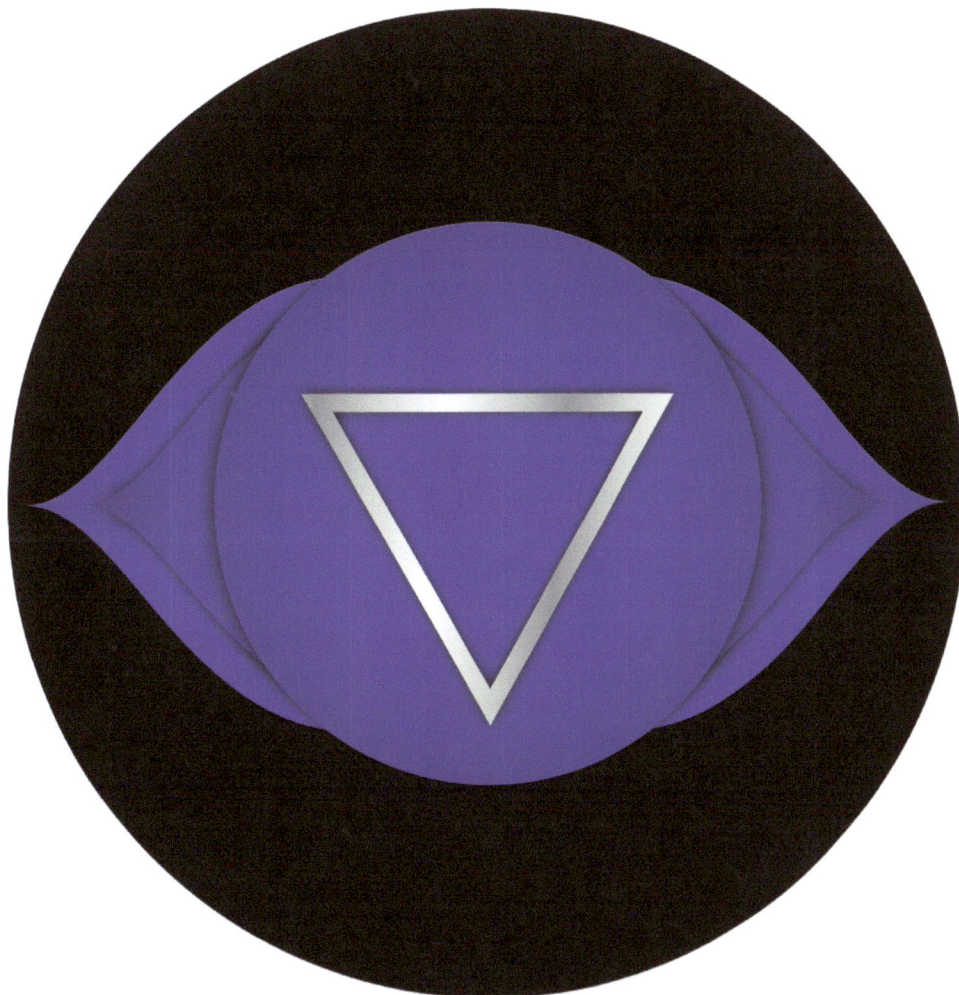

Figure 10. Third Eye Chakra. Image by Peter Lomas from Pixabay

Colour—Purple/Indigo

Element—Light

Seed sound—AUM

Location—between and just above the eyebrows

Sanskrit—Ajna translation—command perceives

The Third Eye Chakra

Physical anatomy—brain, nerves, forehead, eyes, nose, pituitary and pineal glands and the sinuses.

This chakra's colour is purple; however, some describe it as deep indigo. It is sometimes known as the intuition chakra or the Psychic chakra; however, it also governs our imagination, inner visions, and also our conscience and our perception of right and wrong.

It represents your ability to see, use your intuition, use your imagination, remember your dreams, listen to your inner voice, and heed your conscience. The eyes see the material or physical world, Ajna allows us to see other energies, intuition, clairvoyance, imagination, creativity, and visualization. When these two energy channels Ida and Pingala merge with the central energy channel, Sushumna, duality ends.

Blocked symptoms include vision problems, headache, nasal congestion, sinus infection, stroke, brain abnormalities, lack of imagination, difficulty with visualization, rarely remembering your dreams lack of intuition and no sense of inner voice or conscience, you may struggle to have faith in your broader purpose. So, you may feel there's no point in what you're doing, or feel it is insignificant. You might also be struck by your inability to decide. Some people describe this as a feeling of psychological paralysis. If you have a blocked Third Eye Chakra, you might have trouble sleeping, feel clumsy, and struggle to learn new things.

Overloaded symptoms include headache, hyperventilation, brain hemorrhage, hallucinations, psychic abilities that impair normal functioning psychosis, living in a fantasy world, being in your head too much and problems distinguishing dream experiences from actual experiences balancing suggestions include drawing, painting, meditating, visualizing, recording, and interpreting your dreams, paying attention to what you see around you and listening to your intuition.

Yoga poses to aid this chakra—Tadasana, Janu Sirsasana, Uttanasana, Makarasana, and Balasana. Also, practice Seed Mantra Meditation

8.9   The Crown Chakra

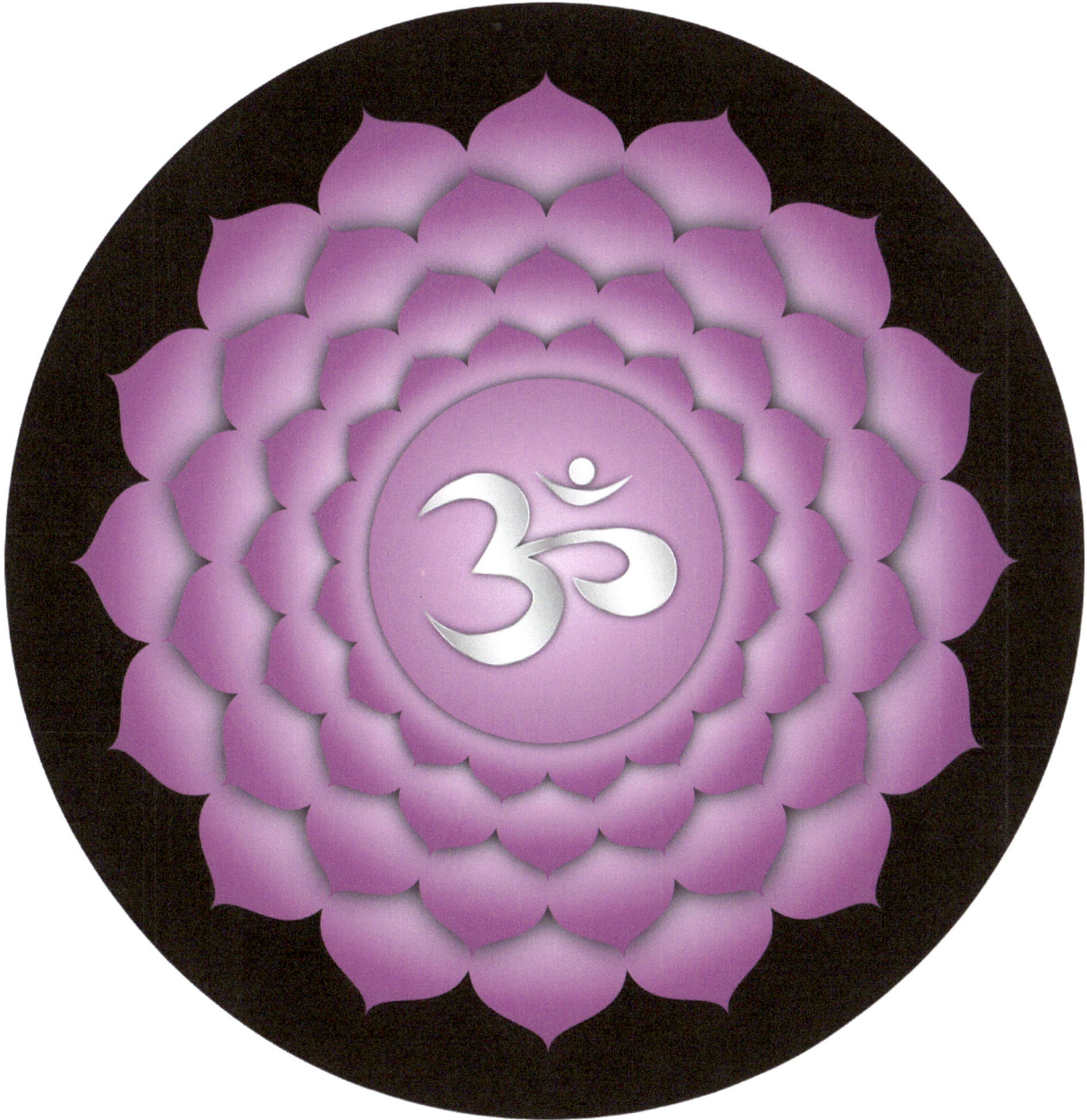

Figure 11. Crown Chakra. Image by Peter Lomas from Pixabay

Colour—White/Purple

Element—thought

Seed sound—AUM

Location—slightly above the crown of the head

Sanskrit—Sahasrara translation—thousand petals "of the lotus flower"

Physical anatomy engaged—the skull, brain, cerebral cortex

The crown chakra is where the "real you" come together because it reflects the human spirit—higher brain function, our connection with the higher power or universal energy, and also our ability to connect to the "big picture" in different aspects of our physical world and how our spirituality and our connectedness are reflected in that. The lotus flower is associated with this chakra, as the actual flower can extend its system through various depths of water and is rooted in deep, murky bottom of ponds, much as we are sometimes mired in the physical elements of this world and yet able to extend ourselves up to the top of the "water" and produce a beautiful result: connection with our higher Self and Universal Energy. This chakra is depicted with the colour white; however, it is sometimes known as purple.

Represents your intellectual ability, your spirituality, your connection to spirit, God, the universe or higher power.

Blocked symptoms are headaches, brain abnormalities, amnesia, feelings of isolation, depression, lack of inspiration and spiritual crisis. You might not see much beauty in the world at all if your Crown Chakra has been disturbed. You may also feel spiritually adrift and experience symptoms of depression. If you're only starting to develop this type of block, you might just notice a decline in overall excitement or motivation. Physically, a blocked Crown Chakra can also occur at the same time as problems with physical coordination or chronic headaches.

Overloaded symptoms are headaches, addiction to spiritual or intellectual practices, out-of-body experiences, dissociation with the body, over—intellectualizing and feeling ungrounded.

Balancing suggestions include meditating, praying, spiritual study, learning new things, grounding, and physical exercises.

Yoga poses to aid this chakra—Ardha Padmasana, Vriksasana, Salamba Sirsasana, Nadi Shodhan Pranayama

9   Aligning Chakras with Yoga Poses

The following matrix is extracted from a table of Yoga poses at:

http://www.liveyoga.nl/yoga-library/sanskrit-dictionary/

Missing Chakra/Pose combinations, Sanskrit, and English translations have been added.

Sanskrit spelling inconsistencies have been corrected.

Sanskrit	English	Chakra	Asanas (Sanskrit)	Poses (English)
Apanasana	knee to chest	Root	Apanasana	Knee to Chest
Janu	knee	Root	Janu Sirsasana	Head to knee forward extension
Salabha	locust	Root	Salabhasana	Locust pose
Setu	Bridge, dam, dike	Root	Setu Bandha Sarvangasana	Bridge pose
Mala	garland	Root	Malasana	Garland poses
Dwipada Pitham	two, both feet	Sacral	Dwipada Pitham	Two-legged Table pose
Salamba Bhujangasana	Sphinx	Sacral	Salamba Bhujangasana	Sphinx Pose
Jathara Parivrtti	belly twist	Sacral	Jathara Parivrtti	Belly Twist
Kapotasana	pigeon	Sacral	Kapotasana	Pigeon Pose
Supta	supine, lying down	Sacral	Supta Virasana, Supta Baddha Konasana, Supta Padangusthasana	Reclining Hero pose, reclining bound angle pose, reclining hand-to-big-toe pose.
Dhanu	bows	Sacral	Dhanurasana, Urdhva Dhanurasana	Bow pose, Upward Bow or Full Wheel pose
Virabhadra	name of a hero in Siva's army	Solar Plexus— Virabhadrasana (I)	Virabhadrasana (I II, III)	Warrior (I II, III)
Navasana	boat	Solar Plexus	Navasana	Boat Pose

Sanskrit	English	Chakra	Asanas (Sanskrit)	Poses (English)
Surya	sun	Solar Plexus	Surya Namaskar	Sun salutation
Tada	mountain	Solar Plexus	Tadasana	Mountain pose
Dhanu	bows	Solar Plexus	Dhanurasana, Urdhva Dhanurasana	Bow pose, Upward Bow or Full Wheel pose
Garuda	eagle	Heart	Garudasana	Eagle poses
Go	cow	Heart	Gomukhasana	Cow face pose
Marjaryasana	Cat	Heart	Marjaryasana	Cat Pose
Matsya	fish	Heart	Matsyasana	Fish pose
Svana	dog	Heart	Urdhva Mukha Svanasana, Adho Mukha Svanasana	Upward facing dog pose, downward facing dog pose
Ustra	camel	Heart	Ustrasana	Camel poses
Bhujanga	serpent	Heart	Bhujangasana	Cobra pose
Matsya	fish	Throat	Matsyasana	Fish pose
Sarva	all	Throat	Salamba Sarvangasana	Supported All limbs pose (shoulder stand)
Viparita Kirani	legs up-the wall	Throat	Viparita Kirani	Legs up-the-wall pose
Jalandhara Bandha	Chin lock	Throat	Jalandhara Bandha	Chin Lock
Bhujanga	serpent	Throat	Bhujangasana	Cobra pose
Tada	mountain	Third Eye	Tadasana	Mountain pose
Tada	mountain	Third Eye	Tadasana	Mountain pose
Parivrtta	revolved, turned around or back	Third Eye	Parivrtta Trikonasana, Parivrtta Parsvakonasana, Parivrtta Janu Sirsasana	Revolving triangle, revolving lateral angle pose, Revolving head-to-knee pose
Balasana	Child	Third Eye	Balasana	Child's Pose

Sanskrit	English	Chakra	Asanas (Sanskrit)	Poses (English)
Uttana	intense stretch	Third Eye	Parsvottanasana, Prasarita Padottanasana, Uttanasana, Paschimottanasana	Intense side stretch pose, Intense standing forward extension, Intense seated forward extension
Makarasana	crocodile	Third Eye	Makarasana	Crocodile Pose
Ardha Padmasana	lotus	Crown	Ardha Padmasana	Half Lotus Pose
Salamba	with support	Crown	Salamba Sirsasana, Salamba Sarvangasana	Supported Head stand, Supported shoulder stand
Vrksa	tree	Crown	Vriksasana, Adho Mukha Vriksasana	Tree pose, Full Arm balance pose
Nadi Shodhan Pranayama	nostril	Crown	Nadi Shodhan Pranayama	Alternate Nostril Breathing

10   Divination

In traditional Tibetan culture, when people begin to suffer from this kind of condition, they ask for a divination. Divination is considered an important means to diagnose the source of energy disturbances and to show what can be done to heal those disturbances. Divination sometimes suggests the need for a soul retrieval. In other cases, even without divination, people may feel that a soul retrieval is warranted.[73]

---

[73] Ibid.

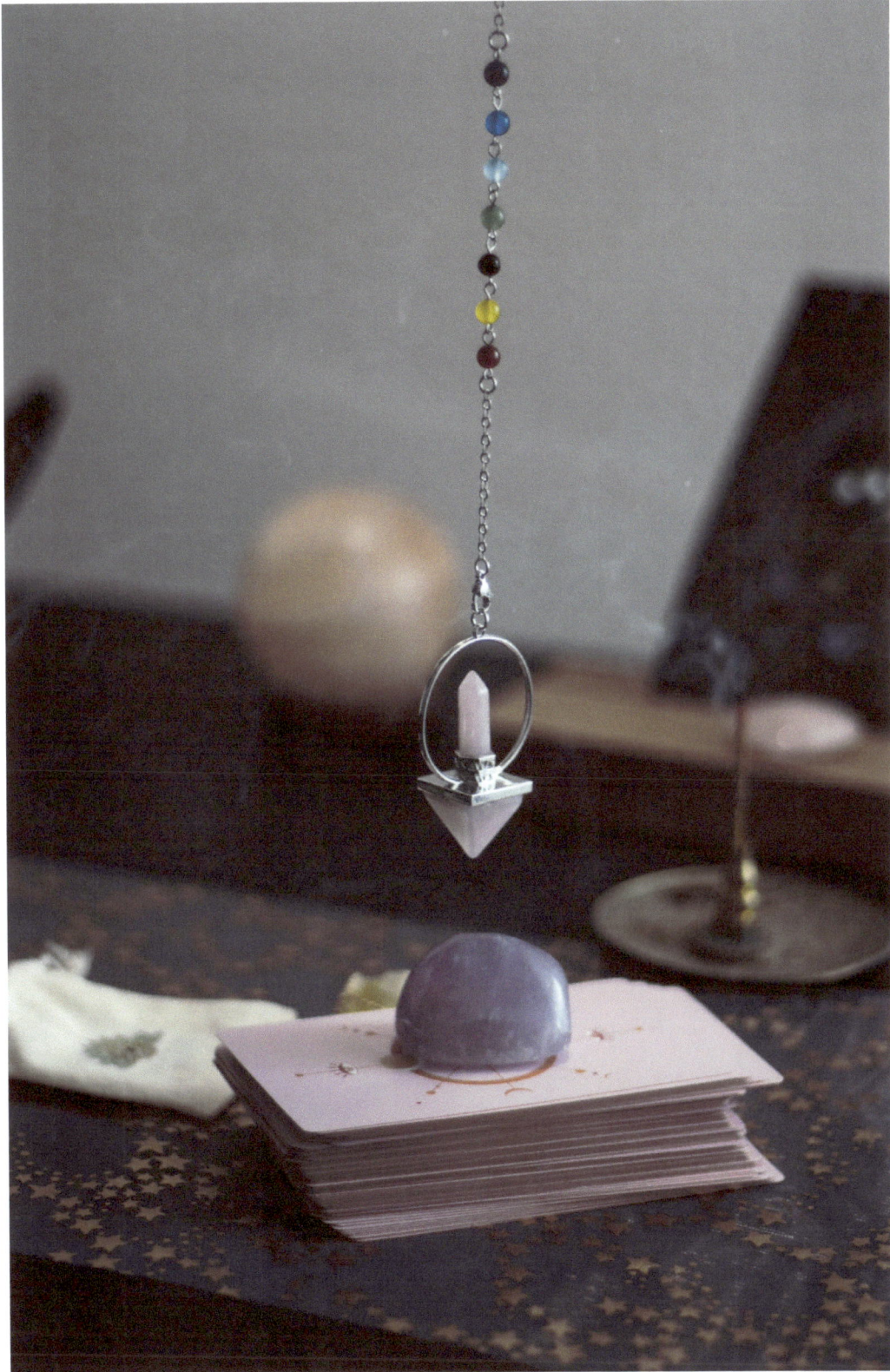

Figure 12. Divination. Photo by Susanna Marsiglia on Unsplash

11   Eight Classes of Being

In Tibet, beings on each class listed below have characteristic appearance, temperaments, and how they relate to humans.

From: The Rigpa Shedra[74] and the Chinese Buddhist Encyclopedia[75]

Name	Tibetan Name	Description
Du	Bdud	The four maras (sometimes also translated as "demons") which create obstacles to practitioners on the spiritual path. It is important to understand that they have no inherent existence and are only created by the mind.
Rakshasa	Srin Po	is a kind of malignant spirit that eats human flesh.
Mamo	Ma Mo	Wrathful feminine deities forming part of Ekadzati's entourage. The mamos are considered being among the main natural forces, which may respond to human misconduct and environmental misuse by creating obstacles and disease.
Naga	Klu	Serpent Spirits live beneath the surface of the earth or in the water, and in trees or rocks, and are believed to be endowed with magical powers and wealth, as well as being responsible for certain types of illnesses (Wyl. klu'i nad) transmitted to humans.
Ging	Ging	Are minor deities who attend to the major deities in some wrathful mandalas. They appear as skeletons who beat a drum, wear a triangular pennant pinned in the middle of their hair, and ear ornaments that look like colourful fans.
Rahula	Sgra gcan 'dzin	The Buddha's son, who also became the tenth of the Sixteen Arhats.
Tsen	btasan	Red spirits that haunt rocks are all male, the spirits of erring monks of earlier times. When they are subdued by a great practitioner, the Tsen often becomes the guardian of temples, shrines, and monasteries. Red offerings are made to them.
YakSha	gnod Sbyin	The name of a broad class of nature spirits, usually benevolent, who are caretakers of the natural treasures hidden in the Earth and tree roots.

Figure 13. From: The Rigpa Shedra and The Chinese Buddhist Encyclopedia

11.1   Four Levels of Guests

In a Shaman's ritual, he/she considers the level of the guests invited to attend a ritual or ceremony; there are guidelines on how to relate to each.

Guest	Description
First Level	• Fully enlightened beings—powerful • Buddha's and Bodhisattvas • Free of Ignorance • They have perfected the five wisdoms • We do not control these guests • We ask for their blessings
Second Level	• Not fully enlightened but powerful

---

[74] Rigpa Wiki, EightClassesofGodsandDemons.
[75] Chinese Buddhist Encyclopedia, EightClassesofGodsandDemons.

Guest	Description
	• From the god realm, they make up the retinue of the major deities' guardians and dharma protectors • They may be from the realm of existence. Such as Angels. • Beings representing the planets and celestial bodies • Second-level guests help with healing. • We treat them with respect and honour them
Third Level	• Beings we have karmic connections with • Karmic connections can mean friends and also enemies—in this lifetime and in past existence. • A connection may also mean something that has to be completed. It could be a duty or obligation to another spirit, by the spirit that is in us. This obligation is often referred to as a Karmic Debt.
Fourth Level	• Guests of compassion • They are weaker than we are. They can benefit from our help. • In the BON shamanic tradition, it is important to develop compassion as a foundation for our practice.

Figure 14. Four Levels of Guests

11.2 Making an offering to the Guests

In all the religious traditions of Tibet, offerings are made to spiritual, non-physical beings.

The Mandala offering is foundational to Bon and four schools of Tibetan Buddhism and is made to the first- and second-level quests.

Other offerings for specific rituals may be Torma, Alcohol, texts, and prayers. These can be especially long prayers or mantras, jewels, and precious stones. Also, acceptable is leftover food, or if food is not prepared or nothing is left over, use of the mind to prepare and gift an imaginary offering is also acceptable.

While we prepare offerings for an important ritual, such as soul retrieval or healing, we should also not forget to make offerings when everything is going well. Maintaining health, harmony, love, and happiness are important things in our lives. Preparing offerings to sustain spirits and our happy state is important. We do not want blockages to appear; we want to ensure we prevent obstacles from manifesting that may block us tomorrow. If nothing more, we are honouring our protectors and guides.

11.3 Chang-Bu Offering

It is a simple offering made of flour and water. It is called Chang-Bu or a fingerprint Torma.

A shaman may make and use it, but this can also be made by yourself.

Mae, the dough so that is not too wet, it must not be sticky. Think of toothpaste; that consistency is an excellent guide for the consistency of the Torma. If you are male, lightly oil the right hand; if female, oil the left hand.

Roll the dough until it is a fat roll.

Press the dough into the palm of the oiled hand sufficiently hard that the tough will take on all the ridges, seams, and channels of the skin. Make sure the palm is covered as well as the fingers and thumb. The five fingers and thumb represent the five elements; we want to capture the creases of the fingers where they flex and bend.

Touch the dough to any part of the body that needs healing. This draws spiritual attention to that spot; prana follows the attention, since mind and prana always move together. With the attention on a single part of the body, sensation in that part increases.

We can experience this by touching any place on our bodies and putting our attention there. When this is done with the change, we use our imagination to draw the illness, trauma, or negativity into the dough.

Try to feel a release in that area of the body. Move the Torma to another part of the body that needs healing. When we have finished, we have a substantial symbol of our illnesses, one that is energetically connected to us; this is offered to the third and fourth guests, the beings who may cause and maintain the illness.

The intent behind the ritual is not only to remove the influence of the spirit from the body, but also to give the spirit something, which is done through the offering. What is given has some of the energetic properties of the illness, but it is now in a purer form that will nourish and satisfy the spirit? When it accepts the offering, it leaves the person whom it has afflicted.

After the ritual is finished, the offering is taken outside and thrown in the direction opposite the individual's birth year sign, the direction, it is believed, in which the negative force is most likely to originate. (If you don't know your sign, refer to the chart at the end of this book.)

Traditionally, after a ritual like this, we look for a dream that signifies success, such as a dream of insects, animals, liquid, or other beings or negative substances coming out of the body.

12   What is a Spirit?

12.1   Etymology

The modern English word "spirit" comes from the Latin spiritus, but also "spirit, soul, courage, vigour," ultimately from a Proto-Indo-European language. The language is the most widely spoken language in the world. It is distinguished from the Latin anima, "soul" (which also derives from an Indo-European root meaning "to breathe," earliest form *h2enh1-). In Greek, this distinction exists between pneuma, "breath, motile air, spirit," and "soul.[76]

The word 'spirit' came into Middle English via Old French. The distinction between soul and spirit developed in the Abrahamic religions and the Arabic and Hebrew languages.

12.2   A Definition

In folk belief, spirit is the vital principle or animating force within all living things. As far back as 1628 and 1633, respectively, both William Harvey and René Descartes speculated that somewhere within the body, in a special locality, there was a 'vital spirit' or 'vital force,' which animated the whole bodily frame, such as the engine in a factory moves the machinery in it. Spirit has frequently been conceived of as a supernatural being, or non-physical entity; for example, a demon, ghost, fairy, or angel. In ancient Islamic terminology, however, a spirit applies only to pure spirits, but not to other invisible creatures, such as jinn, demons, and angels.[77]

The concepts of spirit and soul often overlap, and both are believed to survive bodily death in some religions, and 'spirit' can also have the sense of ghosts, i.e., a manifestation of the spirit of a deceased person. Spirit is also often used to refer to consciousness or personality. [78]

12.3   Dictionary Definition

- The principle of conscious life; the vital principle in humans: animating the body or mediating between body[79]

- the incorporeal part of humans[80]

12.4   Usage

The modern English word 'spirit' comes from the Latin spiritus, but also spirit, soul, courage, and vigour, ultimately from a Proto-Indo-European (s)pays.[81]

Usage[82]	Description[83]

---

[76] Wikipedia, Spirit-Wikipedia.
[77] Ibid.
[78] Ibid.
[79] Dictionary.com, DefinitionofSpirit.
[80] Ibid.
[81] Wikipedia, Spirit.
[82] Ibid.
[83] Ibid.

Usage[82]	Description[83]
Christian Theology	Can use the term 'Spirit' to describe the Holy Spirit.
Christian Science	Christian Science uses 'Spirit' as one of seven synonyms for God, as in: 'Principle; Mind; Soul; Spirit; Life; Truth; Love,,'
Latter-Day Saints	Latter-Day Saint prophet Joseph Smith Jr. taught that the concept of spirit as incorporeal or without substance was incorrect: 'There is no such thing as immaterial matter. All spirit is matter, but it is finer, and can only be discerned by purer eyes." In Mormonism, unlike souls (often regarded as eternal and sometimes believed to pre-exist in the body) a spirit develops and grows as an integral aspect of a living being.
Various forms of Animism	Japan's Shinto and African traditional religion focus on invisible beings that represent or connect with plants, animals, or landforms (kami): translators usually employ the English word "spirit" when trying to express the idea of such entities.
C. G. Jung	In a lecture delivered to the Literary Society of Augsburg, 20 October 1926, on the theme of "Nature and Spirit"

The connection between spirit and life is one of those problems involving factors of such complexity that we have to be on our guard lest we ourselves get caught in the net of words in which we seek to ensnare these great enigmas. For how can we bring into the orbit of our thought those limitless complexities of life, which we call "Spirit" or "Life" unless we clothe them in verbal concepts, themselves mere counters of the intellect? The mistrust of verbal concepts, inconvenient as it is, seems to me to be very much in place in speaking of fundamentals. "Spirit" and "Life" are familiar enough words to us, ancient acquaintances in fact, pawns that for thousands of years have been pushed back and forth on the thinker's chessboard. The problem must have begun in the grey dawn of time, when someone discovered that the living breath which left the body of the dying man in the last death rattle meant more than just air in motion. It can scarcely be an accident onomatopoeic words like ruach (Hebrew), ruch (Arabic), Roho (Swahili) mean "spirit" no less clearly than πνεύμα (pneuma, Greek) and spiritus (Latin). |
| Psychic research | "In all the publications of the Society for Psychical Research, the term "spirit" stands for the personal stream of consciousness whatever else it may ultimately be proved to imply or require" (James H. Hyslop, 1919). |

12.5 Spirit in Christian Theology

The word "spirit" appears either alone or with other words, in the Hebrew Bible Old Testament and the New Testament. Combinations include expressions such as the "Holy Spirit," "Spirit of God," and in Christianity, "Spirit of Christ."[84]

---

84 Wikipedia, Rajneesh.

For most Christian denominations, the Holy Spirit, or Holy Ghost is the third person of the Trinity: The Triune God manifested as God the Father, God the Son, and God the Holy Spirit; each entity itself being God.[85]

The Christian expression of the Holy Spirit emphasizes the moral aspect of the meaning that said in Judaism and this trend has continued into the current period.

The Fruit of the Holy Spirit is a biblical term that sums up nine attributes of a person or community living in accord with the Holy Spirit, according to chapter 5 of the Epistle to the Galatians: "But the Fruit of the Spirit is love, joy, peace, patience, kindness, goodness, faithfulness, gentleness, and self-control.[86]

Christian Theology and structured religious systems are strongly based on a set of codified and documented beliefs and teachings followers are expected to follow. Clergy and religious institutions have been established for worshippers and followers to engage with.

The soul and the spirit are connected, but separable Hebrews 4:12. The soul is the essence of humanity's being; it is who we are. The spirit is the immaterial part of humanity that connects with God.[87]

A centralized authority and an organized, often very wealthy infrastructure accompany these theologies and contain a unique set of rituals, books, and processes for an adherent to follow. From earliest times, these centralized religions have been a centre of political and military power. Even in the 20th and 21st centuries, state entities with enormous economic and military capability continue to exist.

According to historian Oswald Spengler, a distinction between Spirit and Soul has been made by the West and earlier civilizations, which influenced its development. The human spirit can be seen as the heavenly component of humans' nonmaterial makeup—the part that is impersonal or universal. [88]

Some Christians believe the Bible identifies humanity's three basic elements: spirit and soul. They emphasize that the human spirit is the 'real person,' the very core of a person's being, the essential seat of their existence. When a person accepts Jesus Christ as their saviour, it is their human spirit that is transformed as they become "new creatures" in Jesus Christ. The soul, which is the seat of the will, mind and emotions, does not get converted but needs to be renewed daily through the recommended Christian disciplines, such as prayer and reading the Bible. In Islam, Muslims are viewed as having their own spirits, but one that is one with God's spirit. For Spengler, the perception of unity this idea led to important for the emergence of the "consensus" that maintained harmony in Islamic culture, especially during the Golden Age of Islam. [89]

12.6 Spirit, Non-Theological Meaning

The human spirit is a component of human philosophy, psychology, art, and knowledge—the spiritual or mental part of humanity. While the term can be used with the same meaning as "human

---

[85] Ibid.

[86] Bibleinfo.com, WhatIstheFruitoftheSpirit?.

[87]

[88] Wikipedia, HumanSpirit.

[89] Ibid.

soul," the human spirit is sometimes used to refer to the impersonal, universal, or higher component of human nature in contrast to soul or psyche, which can refer to the ego or lower element. The human spirit includes our intellect, emotions, fears, passions, and creativity.[90]

In the models of Daniel A. Helminiak and Bernard Lonergan, human spirit is considered being the mental functions of awareness, insight, understanding, judgment, and other reasoning powers. It is distinguished from the separate component of the psyche, which comprises the entities of emotion, images, memory and personality. [91]

Your spirit is a material part of you; it is non-physical and includes character, personality, and feelings. It is moulded by your experiences and your beliefs. Collectively, these combine to be the external spirit you show to your family, your work colleagues and people at the gym. Your spirit influences your way of thinking, feeling, and behaving, especially if a peer group or required style of behaviour or action is required.

New Age encompasses a very broad range of spiritual or religious beliefs which developed in the Western World during the 1970s. The New Age philosophy is non-unified and includes beliefs and practices from eastern and western religious traditions, as well as a holistic approach to health, motivational and positive psychology research. New Age is so broad because the general development of human understanding started to coalesce across an amazingly wide variety of human experience and empowered people to castoff organized religious structures and organizations. New agers, as they are called, don't limit their belief system to one particular doctrine.

Typically, the belief systems seen under the term New Age adopt a holistic form of divinity that includes but is not limited to the universe, including human beings, and contains a strong emphasis on the spiritual authority of the individual's self. This is accompanied by a common belief in a wide variety of semi-divine non-human entities, such as angels and masters, with whom humans can communicate, particularly through the form of channelling.

Although analytically often considered being religious, those involved typically prefer the designation of spiritual or mind, Body and Spirit and rarely use the term New Age themselves. Many scholars of the subject refer to it as the New Age movement, although others contest this term and suggest that it is better seen as a milieu or zeitgeist.[92]

New Age has antecedents that stretch back to southern Europe in Late Antiquity—between the third and eighth centuries AD. Following the Age of Enlightenment in 18th century Europe, new esoteric ideas developed in response to the development of scientific rationality. Scholars call this new esoteric trend occultism, and this occultism was a key factor in the worldview's development from which the New Age emerged.[93]

New Age literature often refers to benevolent non-human spirits with whom humans can communicate, particularly through the form of channelling. The belief system contains a strong focus on healing using forms of alternative medicine, which includes a strong connection to semi-

---

[90] Ibid.
[91] Ibid.
[92] Wikipedia, DhyanainBuddhism.
[93] Ibid.

divine non-human entities. New Age contains the notion that spirituality and science can be unified. As a result, New Age places Meditation alongside Quantum Physics.

Figure 15. Karma

13 Karma

Karma is the Buddhist term, which literally means doing, action, work, or deed; it also refers to spiritual principal cause and effect where intent and actions of an individual—the cause and its influence the future of that individual—the effect. Good intent and good deeds contribute to good karma and happier rebirths, while bad intent and bad deeds contribute to bad karma and bad rebirths.[94] Understanding karmic action and its result[s] is a foundational concept in Buddhist philosophy. It is an essential aspect of Buddhism.

The philosophy of karma is closely associated with the idea of rebirth in many schools of Indian religions, particularly Hinduism[95], Buddhism[96], Jainism[97] and Sikhism[98] as well as Taoism[99]. In these schools, karma in the present affects one's future in the current life, as well as the nature and quality of future lives—one's samsara.[100] [101]

All Hindu, Jain and Buddhist schools view karma and casualties, or the result, as linked. The actions of a person are carried out, or the intent of a person materially affects the life they lead. The actions and/or intent may be positive or negative. These are purposeful actions and deliberate actions. If the actions are unintentional or accidental, the good, or bad karma arising is not as good or bad as a deliberate or intentional. The karmic effect may be nonexistent or have no effect at all.

In the west, karma is often understood by the simple expression, "what goes around, comes around?" as said by a friend of mine looking at the deliberate keying of the door on her Mercedes. Karmic actions can be thought of as a seedling that will inevitably grow and ripen, and the resulting fruit will either be tasty and delicious, or it will be bitter and tasteless.

So, good karma produces a good effect on the person responsible, while bad karma produces a bad effect —. This effect may be material, moral, or emotional—that is, one's karma affects one's happiness and unhappiness. The effect of karma need not be immediate; the effect of karma can be later in one's current life, and in some schools, it extends to future lives.[102]

The consequence or effects of one's karma can be described in two forms: phalas and samskaras. A phala (literally, fruit or result) is the visible or invisible effect that is typically immediate or within the current life. In contrast, samskaras are invisible effects, produced by the actor because of karma, transforming the agent and affecting his or her ability to be happy or unhappy in this life and future ones. The theory of karma is often presented in the context of samskaras.[103]

Karma of the soul has a significant role to play in reincarnation and the entire cycle of rebirths a soul passes through over and over again. Rebirth is fundamental to Hinduism, Buddhism, Jainism and Sikhism. Reincarnation is a hotly debated subject with some schools of Indian religion. Some

---

[94] https://en.wikipedia.org/wiki/Karma, Karma.

[95] Wikipedia, Hinduism.

[96] Buddhism.

[97] Jainism.

[98] Sikhism.

[99] Taoism.

[100] Ibid.

[101] https://en.wikipedia.org/wiki/Karma, Karma.

[102] Ibid.

[103] Ibid.

accepting Reincarnation and Karma, others not, or some splitting reincarnation and Karma, discarding Reincarnation but holding on to Karma.

In all of this, Tibetan Buddhism agrees with Reincarnation and the role of Karma in the process. This is probably because Tibetan Buddhism adopted and accepted the native Religion of Tibet, Bon.[104] Bon had ingested shamanistic rituals, practices, and oral teachings. It was the dominant religion in Tibet prior to Buddhism's arrival in the eigh[th] century. Today, in 2020, approximately 12.5% of the Tibetan population is followers of Bon.[105] Today, Bon is recognized by the 14th Dali Lama.[106]

Rebirth, or samsara, is the concept that all life forms go through a cycle of reincarnation, which is a series of births and rebirths. The rebirths and consequent life may be in different realms, conditions, or forms. The karma theories suggest that the realm, condition, and form depend on the quality and quantity of karma.[107]

In schools that believe in rebirth, every living being's soul transmigrates (recycles) after death, carrying the seeds of karmic impulses from life just completed, into another life and lifetime of karma. The cycle continues indefinitely, except for those who consciously break this cycle by reaching moksha[108] or nirvana. Those who break the cycle reach the realm of gods, those who don't continue in the cycle.[109]

While ordinary human beings may have trouble judging from direct empirical evidence alone whether or not rebirth actually exists, our inability to perceive its workings cannot conclusively rule out the possibility of its existence. Moreover, our inability to discern something presently doesn't mean that it is forever indiscernible. Empirical evidence may not be taken to serve as the only premise worthy of proving the existence of a certain phenomenon. Besides, we may not have physical evidence for the existence of rebirth, but inasmuch as it is conceivable, it implies that rebirth is more or less reasonable or logical. For example, it seems counterintuitive for the virtuous to die earlier or experience hardship while the wicked enjoy a prosperous life.[110]

For the principle of moral equilibrium to work, therefore, some type of survival beyond the present life should be conceivable. It can further be argued that although ordinary people may not have the perceptual faculties to experience the mechanism of rebirth, it does not necessarily mean that past and future incarnations are imperceptible to evolved beings, such as the yogis of India, who spend a great deal of their lives developing extraordinary faculties. The workings of a cellular phone may be beyond the comprehension of a tiny ant on the ground, yet that does not mean cellular phones don't exist or that such devices may not be perceived by and indeed utilized by evolved beings. Non-experiential claims are not necessarily counter-experiential; that is that one phenomenon goes beyond our experience doesn't mean that it necessarily contradicts our experiences.[111]

---

[104] Wikipedia, Bon.
[105] ReligioninTibet.
[106] Ligmincha International, MessagefromDalaiLama.Pdf.
[107] https://en.wikipedia.org/wiki/Karma, Karma.
[108] Wikipedia, Moksha.
[109] https://en.wikipedia.org/wiki/Karma, Karma.
[110] https://link.springer.com/article/10.1186/s40613-015-0016-2, OntheNaturalizationofKarmaandRebirth.
[111] Ibid.

Bibliography:

Bibleinfo.com. "What Is the Fruit of the Spirit?".

Britannica. "Bardo ThöDol Tibetan Buddhist Text."

Collection, University of California Press eBook. "The Spiritual Quest." (1982 - 2004).

Dictionary, Merriam-Webster. "Definition of Soul by Merriam-Webster."

Dictionary.com. "Definition of Spirit."

———. "Incorporeal."

———. "Spirit Definition of Spirit."

Encyclopedia, Chinese Buddhist. "Eight Classes of Gods and Demons."

English, Longman Dictionary of Contemporary. "Spirit Meaning of Spirit."

Ermakov, Dmitry. "Bo and Bon - Ancient Shamanic Traditions of Siberia and Tibet in Their
        Relation to the Teachings of a Central Asian Buddha."

GotQuestions.org. "What Is the Difference between the Soul and Spirit of Man?".

Honolulu, Master Sha Tao Center. "Open Spiritual Channels Soul Language and Translation -
        Honolulu Tao Healing Soul Healing Energy Healing Master Sha."

http://donlehmanjr.com/. "The Tibetan Book of the Dead.Pdf."

http://healerofheartsandminds.com. "Reincarnation, Past Lives, Suffering and the Bible, a
        Shaman's Views."

https://en.wikipedia.org/wiki/Karma. "Karma."

https://en.wikipedia.org/wiki/The_City_of_God. "The City of God."

https://link.springer.com/article/10.1186/s40613-015-0016-2. "On the Naturalization of
        Karma and Rebirth."

https://lissarankin.com, Lissa Rankin. "20 Diagnostic Signs That You're Suffering from Soul
        Loss."

https://www.wisdomlib.org. "Antarabhava, AntarāBhava 2 Definitions."

International, Ligmincha. "Message from Dalai Lama.Pdf."

Lionsroar.com. "The Four Points of Letting Go in the Bardo."

Philosophy, Stanford Encyclopedia of. "Descartes and the Pineal Gland."

Rinpoche, Tenzin Wangyal. "Soul Retrieval and Related Ideas."

———. "Tibetan Soul Retrieval."

Theinnervoyage.com. "Soul Retrieval."

Wiki, Rigpa. "Eight Classes of Gods and Demons."

Wikipeda. "History of the Location of the Soul."

Wikipedia. "Animal."

———. "Animism."

———. "Ascended Master."

———. "Bardo."

———. "Bardo Thodol."

———. "Bon."

———. "Buddhism."

———. "Carl Jung."

———. "Carol Zaleski."

———. "Cellular Respiration."

———. "Dhyana in Buddhism."

———. "Dissociation Psychology."

———. "Dzogchen."

———. "Hinduism."

———. "Human Body."

———. "Human Spirit."
———. "Jainism."
———. "Moksha."
———. "Rajneesh."
———. "Reincarnation."
———. "Religion in Tibet."
———. "Robert Thurman."
———. "Sikhism."
———. "Skandha."
———. "Sogyal Rinpoche."
———. "Soul."
———. "Spirit."
———. "Spirit - Wikipedia."
———. "Taoism."
Woolger, Dr. Roger J. "Beyond Death- Transition and the Afterlife."
www.rigpawiki.org. "Emptiness."
———. "Nyingma Buddhism."

www.ingramcontent.com/pod-product-compliance
Lightning Source LLC
Chambersburg PA
CBHW060859270326
41935CB00003B/30